UNDERSTANDING INSULIN ACTION:
Principles and Molecular Mechanisms

J. ESPINAL, B.Sc., D.Phil
Head of Diabetes Research Section
Department of Endocrinology, Glaxo Research Laboratories
Research Triangle Park, North Carolina, USA

ELLIS HORWOOD LIMITED
Publishers · Chichester

First published in 1989 by
ELLIS HORWOOD LIMITED
Market Cross House, Cooper Street,
Chichester, West Sussex, PO19 1EB, England
The publisher's colophon is reproduced from James Gillison's drawing of the ancient Market Cross, Chichester.

Distributors:

Australia and New Zealand:
JACARANDA WILEY LIMITED
GPO Box 859, Brisbane, Queensland 4001, Australia

Europe and Africa:
JOHN WILEY & SONS LIMITED
Baffins Lane, Chichester, West Sussex, England

North and South America and Canada:
CHAPMAN AND HALL, INC.
29 West 35th Street
New York, NY 10001–2291

South-East Asia
JOHN WILEY & SONS (SEA) PTE LIMITED
37 Jalan Pemimpin # 05–04
Block B, Union Industrial Building, Singapore 2057

Indian Subcontinent
WILEY EASTERN LIMITED
4835/24 Ansari Road
Daryaganj, New Delhi 110002, India

© **1989 J. Espinal/Ellis Horwood Limited**

Espinal, J.
Understanding insulin action: principles and molecular mechanisms.
(Ellis Horwood series in biotechnology)

CIP catalogue record for this book is available from the British Library

Library of Congress card no. also available

ISBN 0–7458–0473-X (Ellis Horwood Limited)
ISBN 0–412–02661–3 (Chapman and Hall, Inc.)

Typeset in Times by Ellis Horwood Limited
Printed in Great Britain by The Camelot Press, Southampton

327210

UNDERSTANDING INSULIN ACTION:
Principles and Molecular Mechanisms

Ellis Horwood books in the
BIOLOGICAL SCIENCES
General Editor: Dr ALAN WISEMAN, University of Surrey, Guildford
Series in BIOTECHNOLOGY
Series Editor: Dr ALAN WISEMAN, Senior Lecturer in the Division of
Biochemistry, University of Surrey, Guildford

Aitken, J.	**Handbook of Enzyme Active Site Identification***
Ambrose, E.J.	**The Nature and Origin of the Biological World**
Austin, B. & Brown, C.M.	**Microbial Biotechnology: Freshwater and Marine Environments***
Berkeley, R.C.W., *et al.*	**Microbial Adhesion to Surfaces**
Bertoncello, I.	**Human Cell Cultures for Screening Anti-Cancer Rays***
Blackburn, F. & Knapp, J.S.	**Agricultural Microbiology***
Bowen, W.R.	**Membrane Separation Processes***
Bubel, A. & Fitzsimons, C.	**Microstructure and Function of Cells**
Clarke, C.R. & Moos, W. H.	**Drug Discovery Technologies***
Cooke, N.	**Potassium Channels***
Corkill, J.A.	**Clinical Biochemistry:**
	The Analysis of Biologically Important Compounds and Drugs*
Crabbe, M.J.C.	**Enzyme Biotechnology and Protein Engineering**
Crabbe, M.J.C.	**Kinetics of Enzymes***
Denyer, S. & Baird, R.	**Handbook of Microbiological Control***
Dolly, J.O.	**Neurotoxins in Neurochemistry**
Espinal, J.	**Understanding Insulin Action:**
	Principles and Molecular Mechanisms
Eyzaguirre, J.	**Chemical Modification of Enzymes**
Eyzaguirre, J.	**Human Biochemistry and Molecular Biology**
Ferencik, M.	**Immunochemistry***
Fish, N.M.	**Computer Applications in Fermentation Technology***
Francis, J.L.	**Haemostasis and Cancer***
Gacesa, P. & Russell, N.J.	**Pseudomonas Infection and Alginates:**
	Structures, Properties and Functions in Pathogenesis*
Gemeiner, P. *et al.*	**Enzyme Engineering***
Harding, J.	**Biochemistry and Pharmacology of Cataract Research:**
	Drug Therapy Approaches*
Horobin, R.W.	**Understanding Histochemistry:**
	Selection, Evaluation and Design of Biological Stains
Hudson, M.J. & Pyle, P.L.	**Separations for Biotechnology, Vol 2***
Hughes, J.	**The Neuropeptide CCK***
Jordan, T.W.	**Fungal Toxins and Chemistry***
Junter, G.A.	**Electrochemical Detection Techniques in the Applied Biosciences:**
	Vol. 1: Analysis and Clinical Applications
	Vol. 2: Fermentation and Bioprocess Control, Hygiene and Environmental Sciences
Kennedy, J.F. & White, C.A.	**Bioactive Carbohydrates**
Krcmery, V.	**Antibiotic and Chemotherapeutic Compounds***
Krstulovic, A. M.	**Chiral Separations by HPLC**
Palmer, T.	**Understanding Enzymes, 2nd Edition**
Paterson, R.	**Biological Applications of Membranes**
Reizer, J. & Peterkofsky, A.	**Sugar Transport and Metabolism in Gram-positive Bacteria**
Russell, N. J.	**Microbes and Temperature***
Scragg, A.H.	**Biotechnology for Engineers:**
	Biological Systems in Technological Processes
Sikyta, B.	**Methods in Industrial Microbiology**
Sluyser, M.	**Molecular Biology of Cancer Genes**
Sluyser, M. & Voûte, P.A.	**Molecular Biology and Genetics of Childhood Cancers:**
	Approaches to Neuroblastoma
Verrall, M.S.	**Discovery and Isolation of Microbial Prodoucts**
Verrall, M.S. & Hudson, M.J.	**Separations for Biotechnology**
Webb, C. & Mavituna, F.	**Plant and Animal Cells: Process Possibilities**
Winkler, M.	**Biochemical Process Engineering***
Wiseman, A.	**Handbook of Enzyme Biotechnology, 2nd Edition**
Wiseman, A.	**Topics in Enzyme and Fermentation Biotechnology Vols. 1, 2, 4, 6, 8**
Wiseman, A.	**Enzyme Induction, Mutagen Activation and Carcinogen Testing in Yeast**
Wiseman, A.	**Genetically Engineered Proteins and Enzymes from Yeasts***

* *In preparation*

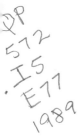

Table of contents

*To the people most dear to me:
my parents, my wife Angela,
and our daughter Lucia.*

Preface

Every year between three and four hundred papers are published on the topic of insulin action. This extraordinary publication rate prevents any author from including an exhaustive bibliography in any review or book. Perhaps due to this there is no single text that attempts to cover the effects and the mechanism of action of insulin. This book is such an attempt. I intend to present a review of the physiological effects of insulin, the pathology of defects in the action of insulin, and the current views on the mechanism of action of this hormone. I make no apology for the fact that the bibliography will not be extensive and that the amount of experimental detail and data discussed will be kept to a relevant minimum. This book is not intended for the expert in the field, but for the second- or third-year undergraduate and graduate student of medicine, biochemistry, physiology or related disciplines, and will be valuable as a reference source for research workers. The book is presented as a guide, a summary of the ideas and facts; it will present a reader with a foretaste of a fascinating and ever-changing field. I have attempted to be up-to-date with published research work. Any significant contributions to the field not included in the first draft have been added as footnotes. I assume a basic knowledge of the metabolic pathways of carbohydrates, fats and proteins. No details of the regulation of a given metabolic pathway are given unless they are pertinent to the effects of insulin. The reader will be referred to papers, reviews or textbooks where appropriate.

The book is divided into seven chapters. I introduce the topics by discussing the discovery of insulin in 1922 and the clinical importance of this major finding. I also present the notion that, whilst insulin is one of the best known and characterized proteins, we still do not know its mechanism of action. Insulin works, but how and why? In attempting to take the reader through this mystery (it is almost a whodunnit!) it is essential to introduce the main characters. Thus, in Chapter 2 the chemistry, synthesis and secretion of insulin are discussed. The reason for the importance of insulin lies in the fact that its absence or failure to act results in one of the leading causes of death in Western countries: diabetes. In order to understand the disease and why insulin is so important, I discuss in Chapter 3 the metabolic effects of insulin and present the molecular basis of these effects. The clinical profile of diabetes is also included in order to give the reader a notion of the severity of the disease and of the role that the mechanism of action of insulin may play in its pathology.

Having introduced the characters and the setting, it is time to get into the mystery! In Chapter 4, the molecular mechanisms whereby insulin regulates the activity of its target enzymes (identified in Chapter 3) are discussed in detail. Chapter 5 discusses our current knowledge of the insulin receptor protein itself and its role in the mechanism of action of insulin. Chapter 6 is concerned with how hormones and other agonists communicate their message to the inside of a cell. The two familiar systems of transmembrane signalling (cAMP and inositol phosphates) are presented and the effects of insulin on both discussed. A third signalling system has been discovered in the last couple of years, which appears to be involved mainly with insulin. The inositol phosphoglycan second messenger is presented and its role in insulin action discussed.

Finally, the conclusion to the mystery has to be presented. Unfortunately, there is no butler to blame! In a review I wrote over a year ago, I described insulin as the elusive Pimpernel of endocrinology. This fascinating hormone continues to be just that. Chapter 7 summarizes what has been presented in previous chapters and attempts to gather it all into one unifying hypothesis of insulin action, perhaps a foolish idea! I finish the chapter by discussing any possible therapeutic implications of our current understanding of insulin action. The opinions expressed in this book represent my views and do not reflect the opinions, interests or reasearch directions of my company, Glaxo Inc.

I wish to thank the two persons who have taught me my profession and are responsible for my interest in the area of diabetes: Dr Eric A. Newsholme, with whom I worked for my D.Phil., and Sir Philip J. Randle, FRS, in whose department I was a research fellow. I also wish to thank Dr Pedro Cuatrecasas, Senior Vice-President of Research at Glaxo Inc., for his critical assessment of this manuscript, enthusiasm and support.

The final thanks have to be for my wife, Angela Rae, for her constant encouragement, support and inspiration.

List of abbreviations

This list includes only those abbreviations that have not been referred to in the text and which are frequently used.

ACTH:	Adrenocorticotrophic hormone
cAMP:	Cyclic 3′, 5′-adenosine monophosphate
AMP:	Adenosine monophosphate
ADP:	Adenosine diphosphate
ATP:	Adenosine trisphosphate
CSF:	Colony-stimulating factor
EGF:	Epidermal growth factor
IGF-I:	Insulin-like growth factor-I
IGF-II:	Insulin-like growth factor-II
PDGF:	Platelet-derived growth factor

1

Introduction

In the introduction to one of the few books in the area of insulin action, the editor confesses to have accepted the invitation to edit the book in a moment of weakness. I can not only sympathize with his feelings but add that my weaknesses are obviously far greater because I am attempting to address a different readership. I hope that the reader will bear with my attempts at writing general prose in guiding him (or her) through the book and trying to excite him about this engaging topic in medical research, the action of insulin.

Diabetes is one of the more familiar diseases; that is, the general public has, by and large, heard of it and it is associated in their minds with insulin. I wish to entice the reader to find out why diabetes occurs and why insulin is the only therapy for those diabetics who lack it. Specifically, I wish to take the reader through a journey starting in the pancreas, where insulin is made and from where it is secreted, and ending in the molecular mechanisms involved in the effects of insulin on the metabolic pathways of the body. As with all journeys it has a point of departure, and, in my view, what better than what has been described as 'the most dramatic event in the history of the treatment of disease' (Bliss, 1982) and 'one of the greatest achievements of modern medicine': the discovery of insulin. In his work on this topic, *The discovery of insulin*, the historian Michael Bliss points out that the magnitude of the discovery can only be comprehended by looking at photographs of patients before and after insulin treatment. In Bliss's words: 'Those who watched the first starved, sometimes comatose, diabetics receive insulin and return to life saw one of the greatest miracles of modern medicine. They were present at the closest approach to the resurrection of the body that our secular society can achieve...'. What follows is a brief summary of the events leading to the discovery of insulin. For a full and authoritative account, the reader is not only referred to, but encouraged to read, Bliss's book.

1.1 A SHORT ACCOUNT OF THE DISCOVERY OF INSULIN

Prior to the discovery of insulin in 1922, diabetics died a slow and progressively weakening death. The word diabetes comes from the Greek word meaning siphon, and is attributed to Arateus of Capadoccia, who in the first century A.D. provided the somewhat colourful description of diabetes as the 'melting down of the flesh and limbs into urine'. When physicians in the seventeenth century noticed that both the urine and the serum of diabetics were sweet, the word 'mellitus' (for honey) was added to the term. By the turn of this century it was possible to diagnose the disease reasonably accurately, but it was impossible to treat it. Diabetics suffered a progressive weight-loss and wasting, were liable to infections and prone to gangrene, non-healing wounds, blindness and a clinical prognosis that was always poor. Starvation, low- or no-carbohydrate diets and other extreme dietary manipulations became standard treatments (advocated by such famous physicians as Frederick Allen and Elliot Joslin), which, when successful, merely delayed the terminal outcome.

The pioneering work of the French physician Claude Bernard at the end of the nineteenth century indicated the primary role of the liver in carbohydrate metabolism and showed that this tissue was able to produce glucose from substrates obtained from digestion of food. Bernard's *Leçons sur le diabète* (1877) is still providing food for thought for scientists today (see Chapter 3). His work pointed towards the liver as one of the important organs in diabetes.

Simultaneous with these studies were the observations obtained in autopsy that in diabetics there was extensive damage to the pancreas. Diabetes was beginning to be ascribed to disease of the pancreas by the end of the last century. In 1889, Minkowski and von Mering performed their now famous experiment of removing the pancreas from a dog and producing sysmptoms like those observed in diabetic patients. Their experiment was all the more remarkable for being one of the few successful total pancreatectomies of the time. Clearly, there was something in the pancreas that was responsible for controlling blood sugar. In their own words: '. . .diabetes as observed after complete removal of the pancreas is exclusively attributed to a stopping of the function in that organ which is necessary for sugar metabolism. We have dealt here with a function of the pancreas hitherto completely unknown.' (von Mering & Minkowski, 1889.)

Ligation of the ducts leading from the pancreas to the duodenum resulted in gastric misfunction but not diabetes. The pancreas therefore had two functions: production of an 'external' secretion consisting of the digestive juices, and of an 'internal' secretion which somehow regulated carbohydrate metabolism. These two functions seemed to correlate with the two types of cells that Langerhans had identified in the pancreas. The acini secrete pancreatic juices and are predominant across the pancreas. Langerhans' discovery was the identification of some cells that appeared to float like islands in amongst the acini. These cells were later named by others the islets of Langerhans and identified with the function of producing the 'internal' secretion responsible for carbohydrate regulation.

Over the thirty or so years following Minkowski and von Mering's experiment, many researchers attempted to administer pancreatic extracts to diabetic subjects hoping that whatever the 'internal' secretion of the pancreas was, it would alleviate their diabetes. It is interesting to note that many attempts were halted because of the coma that developed in some cases following administration; it is likely that these were observations of hypoglycaemia achieved by the presence of insulin in the samples. Of all the attempts at extraction of the 'internal' secretion of the pancreas, perhaps the closest to success was that of a German physician, G. L. Zueler, who actually treated some patients with his extracts, even managing to bring one of them out of a diabetic coma. Two other important scientists who paved the way for the discovery of insulin in 1922 were the American E. L. Scott, who had been partially successful in extracting insulin from the pancreas with alcohol, and N. C. Paulesco, a Romanian who made a pancreatic extract that lowered plasma glucose in dogs and who is claimed by some as the first discoverer of insulin.

In 1920 a paper appeared in the medical literature by Moses Barron on a strange case in which a pancreatic stone had blocked the main pancreatic duct. Whilst the acini atrophied, the islets of Langerhans did not. This gave a Canadian physician, Frederick Banting, an idea of how to obtain the 'internal' secretion of the pancreas separate from the 'external' secretion: if the duct were ligated, the acini would degenerate leaving the islets behind. Banting suggested the idea to J. J. R. Macleod, Professor of Physiology at the University of Toronto. Macleod was critical of the idea and unconvinced of its experimental usefulness but he agreed to make facilities available for Banting to perform his experiments. Banting arrived in Toronto in May 1921 and was introduced by Macleod to Charles Best who was to work as Banting's assistant. Banting and Best thus set out to work on a series of experiments that would immortalize their names in medical history. In February 1922 they published a paper in the *Journal of Laboratory and Clinical Medicine* on their first 75 injections of pancreatic extracts to pancreatomized dogs, claiming a high success rate in lowering blood sugar.

Banting and Best continued their work by attempting to improve the production of an effective extract. Macleod's suggestion of using alcohol yielded positive results even in fresh, non-ligated pancreas. At this point, J. B. Collip, a biochemist from the University of Alberta, joined the team. Towards the end of 1922 Collip had made several ground-breaking observations: firstly he showed that the alcohol extract caused an increase in glycogen formation in the liver of a diabetic dog; secondly he showed that the extract also caused the disappearance of ketone bodies from the urine of diabetic dogs; and finally he was able to make some further refinements to the method of producing the extract.

On January 11, 1922, the first clinical test of the extract was performed. It was injected into a 14-year-old diabetic, Leonard Thompson. The results were not encouraging: the fall in blood glucose was not very marked and ketones were still present in urine. A few days afterwards Collip made the most significant improve-ment in the purification: he discovered that, at an alcohol concentration of approxi-mately 90%, the active principle in the extract could precipitate out. Twelve days after his first injection, Leonard Thompson received an injection of Collip's new extract. His blood sugar level became normal and his ketonuria was eliminated. The boy received injections of the extract for several days and his condition improved. The Toronto team presented their work at the meeting of the Association of American Physicians in Washington, D.C. on May 23, 1922, to a standing ovation.

Controversy has always surrounded the discovery of insulin, particularly because of the disagreements and antagonisms between the members of the Toronto team over the credit of the inception of the idea. In the case of the discovery of insulin, however, credit must go to all. As Bliss points out, insulin was discovered by a team led by Macleod, working on a project initiated by Banting with Best, and where

Collip had made the most significant technical achievements, not by Banting and Best alone. The Nobel Prize was awarded to Banting and Macleod on October 25, 1923. Banting announced immediately that he was sharing his prize with Best; Macleod did the same with Collip. History has honoured all four.

1.2   AN OVERVIEW OF INSULIN ACTION AND DIABETES

The discovery of insulin was a miraculous event for the diabetics, for whom the disease was an effective sentence of death. Insulin treatment of diabetics resulted in a couple of ironies. Instead of 'curing' diabetes — as it had been initially hoped — the number of diabetics worldwide increased because of their longer life-expectancy and transmission of their disease to their progeny. Also, as the life-expectancy of diabetics increased (as much as 25-fold!), the long-term complications of diabetes came into effect. Today diabetics still have a lower life-expectancy then non-diabetics due to renal failure, cardiovascular disease, blindness and other complications. Joslin is said to have commented that insulin eliminated coma as the cause of death in diabetes but opened the way to renal or cardiovascular complications.

It is worth pointing out very briefly that not all diabetics require insulin to survive. In fact, the insulin-dependent diabetics (or juvenile-onset patients) comprise only about 10% of all diabetics. The aetiology of type I diabetes is complex and not fully understood, but the essential point to remember is that in this disease there is a destruction of the pancreatic B-cell. Therefore, patients are unable to synthesize or secrete insulin. The vast majority of diabetics, however, can control their disease with diet alone, or diet plus oral hypoglycaemic agents (not known in Banting's time). In these patients (maturity-onset or non-inuslin-dependent diabetics) the defect resides in the inability of insulin to be synthesized and secreted in response to glucose to the same extent as in non-diabetic controls, and/or to exert its effects in target tissues. These issues are considered in detail in Chapter 3.

Whilst pure preparations of insulin were being used to treat diabetics, it took many years for scientists to work out that insulin was a protein. As it happens insulin was also the first protein whose structure was completely sequenced (Ryle *et al.*, 1955) — a discovery that gave Frederick Sanger a Nobel Prize in 1959 — and the first to be chemically synthesized (Katsoyannis *et al.*, 1963). The crystal structure of insulin was one of the first protein structures to be determined (see, for instance, Blundell *et al.*, 1972). To this impressive list of 'firsts' for insulin one has to add another path-breaking discovery: human insulin was the first protein to be commercially produced by recombinant DNA technology for clinical use (Goeddel *et al.*, 1979). However, more than sixty years after its discovery and in spite of the impressive array of scientific breakthroughs associated with insulin we are still in the dark where the mechanism of action of this hormone is concerned. Insulin continues to be the elusive Pimpernel of endocrinology. This is the topic and the purpose of this book: to give an account of the current views concerning the question of how insulin works. It is practically impossible to summarize the various hypotheses on this area in a couple of paragraphs, but in order to give the reader a flavour of things to come an overview follows.

Insulin is a polypeptide hormone, synthesized in and secreted from the pancreas in response to changes in the plasma levels of glucose. The major sites of action of insulin are liver, muscle and adipose tissue, where insulin — as an anabolic hormone — promotes the synthesis of storage fuels such as glycogen, fat or protein. In addition, and as one of the ways in which it promotes these effects, insulin stimulates the uptake of glucose by peripheral tissues, thereby regulating the plasma levels of glucose. This stimulation is observed only in muscle and adipose tissue; no other tissues respond to insulin in this way. The molecular mechanisms regulating these processes are complex but can be placed into three categories. Insulin promotes the dephosphorylation of key regulatory enzymes, or in some cases it stimulates their phosphorylation; the interconversion between different phosphorylation states leads to the activation or inhibition of enzymes involved. In addition, insulin promotes the movement of transporter or receptor proteins — such as the glucose transporter — to the plasma membrane. These issues are discussed in Chapters 3 and 4.

Insulin produces all of its effects without crossing the plasma membrane. Instead, it binds to highly specific receptors localized in the plasma membrane of most cell types. Binding to the receptor results in transmission of the signal to the target enzymes involved in the regulation of metabolic processes. The receptor is composed of two different subunits (α and β) and exhibits a tyrosine kinase activity in one of the subunits (β). Although no intracellular targets of physiological relevance have been identified for the tyrosine kinase, it is generally agreed that the autophosphorylation of the insulin receptor at tyrosine residues in response to insulin is the first absolute requirement for the action of the hormone (see Chapter 5).

The signals involved in transmitting the message could be many and, in spite of a constant search, a second messenger for insulin has proved elusive. Insulin differs from all other hormones in that it does not share the common signalling pathways that involve either cAMP-mediated events or inositol trisphosphate-induced mobilization of calcium. One promising candidate for a second messenger role in the action of insulin has emerged in the last few years: the inositol phosphoglycans (Chapter 6). Whether these structures are proved to be of physiological importance only time will tell.

On the basis of the above, it is possible to unify these concepts into one single hypothesis of insulin action, and this is attempted in the last chapter of the book. I hope that this text will stimulate the imagination of younger students to unravel the questions posed in each of the chapters.

REFERENCES

Banting, F. & Best, C. (1922) *J. Lab. Clin. Med.* **8**(5), 256–257.
Bernard, C. (1877) *Leçons sur le diabète*, J. B. Baillière et fils, Paris.
Bliss, M. (1982) *The discovery of insulin*, University of Chicago Press, Chicago.
Blundell, T. L., Dodson, G. G., Hodsgkin, D. C. & Mercola, D. A. (1972) *Adv. Protein Chem.* **26**, 279.
Goeddel, D. V., Kleid, D. G., Bolivar, F., Heyneker, H. L., Yansura, D. G., Crea, A., Hirose, T., Kraszewski, A., Itakura, K. & Riggs, A. D. (1979) *Proc. Natl. Acad. Sci. USA* **76**, 106–110.
Katsoyannis, P. G., Tometsko, A., Fukuda, K. (1963) *J. Am. Chem. Soc.* **85**, 2863.
Ryle, A. P., Sanger, F., Smith, L. F. & Kitai, R. (1955) *Biochem. J.* **60**, 541–546.
von Mering, J. & Minkowski, O. (1889) *Arch. Exp. Path. Pharmacol.* **26**, 371–387.

2

Insulin: chemistry, synthesis and secretion

Any attempt at understanding the aetiology and pathophysiology of diabetes, particularly type II or non-insulin-dependent diabetes, and at evaluating therapeutic strategies to treat the disease must start with a knowledge of the structure of insulin and its related chemistry. Significant consideration must be given to how insulin is synthesized in, and secreted from, the pancreas. The latter topics are of less relative importance with insulin-dependent or type I diabetes since the destruction of the β-cell is the pathological defect in this condition. In type II diabetes, the ability of the pancreas to synthesize and secrete insulin is maintained. In fact, the ability to secrete insulin in response to such secretagogues as arginine is the same as in controls. However, the response to glucose is considerably decreased. These observations emphasise the need for consideration of the above topics in therapeutic evaluation.

This chapter summarizes three different areas of research where many excellent reviews exist. In each case, a summary of the field is presented and the reader will be referred to the relevant reviews where appropriate.

2.1 THE INSULIN MOLECULE

2.1.1 Primary structure and evolutionary conservation

Insulin was the first protein whose sequence was determined (Ryle *et al.*, 1955). Sanger and co-workers established that the insulin molecule consists of two peptide chains, A and B, linked by two disulphide bridges (Fig. 2.1). Insulin is not synthesized as two separate chains but as a single-chain polypeptide (proinsulin) folded in such a way that its two ends are linked by disulphide bridges between cysteine residues; the connecting peptide, or C-peptide, extends from the amino terminus of the B-chain to the carboxy terminus of the A-chain. Proteolytic cleavage leads to the formation of the insulin molecule and a separate C-peptide (Fig. 2.2).

The A-chain, so called for its relatively acidic nature, has 21 amino acids and an internal disulphide bridge. The more basic B-chain has 30 amino acids. These figures correspond to the numbers of amino acids found in most mammalian insulins. Some hystricomorph insulins, such as that of coypu, have 22 amino acids in the A-chain and

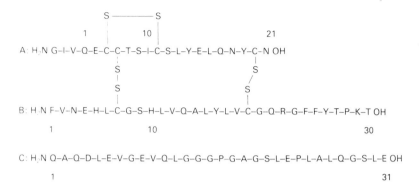

Fig. 2.1 — The primary structure of insulin. A and B are the respective chains in the insulin molecule; C is the connecting peptide. The C-peptide (or C-chain) C-terminal Gln is connected to the N-terminal Gly of the A-chain by an Arg-Lys dipeptide link. At the other end (N-terminal Glu to C-terminal Thre of B-chain) the link is Arg-Arg. These links are susceptible to protease cleavage. Boxed regions denote conserved residues. The single letter amino acid code has been used in this figure. Disulphide bridges are shown by -S-S-.

29 in the B-chain. In fact, one of the most remarkable features of the insulin molecule is its extraordinarily high degreee of evolutionary conservation. Thus, the dual-chain structure and all the disulphide bridges (three in total: two linking the A- and B-chains and an internal one in the A-chain) are conserved in all the different species in insulin that have been isolated and studied. The conservation of this basic structural framework must imply a functional requirement for biological activity. Thus, if the disulphide bridges are broken by reduction there is a total loss of activity.

The evolutionary conservation of insulin's structure goes even further in that the primary amino acid sequences also differ very little. For example, pork and human insulins differ only by one amino acid residue in the B-chain: B30 is alanine and threonine respectively. Further, the amino acid sequence of the insulin molecule of the most primitive vertebrate alive, the cyclotome hagfish, differs from that of pork by only 18 residues and has maintained the basic structure. This degree of conservation is remarkably high for any protein, and must suggest both the physiological importance of insulin overall, and the structural requirements for its activity. Furthermore, examination of the amino acid sequences of the A- and B-chains across species reveal several invariant regions, as shown in Fig. 2.1. Apart from the six cysteine residues, located always in the same positions, three or four other regions are of interest: the first three amino acids at the amino terminus of the A-chain; a region of eight amino acids in the middle of the B-chain; the carboxy-terminal seven amino acids of the B-chain and the three equivalent ones of the A-chain. Let us examine each of these regions of conservation separately and discuss their possible roles in the biological activity of insulin.

The first amino acid of the A-chain, A1 Gly, is always conserved. It is thought that the positive charge of this residue may be important in the binding of insulin to its receptor. Thus, substitution by neutral residues leads to loss of activity.

Continuing in the A-chain, the carboxy-terminal three amino acids, A19 Tyr,

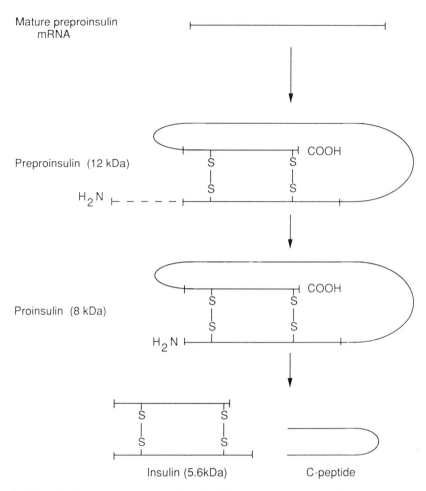

Fig. 2.2 — The biosynthetic pathways of insulin. Schematic representation of cleavage events in the biosynthesis of insulin. The lines represent the amino acids of RNA sequences.

A20 Cys and A21 Asn are always conserved as well. Modifications in these residues results in loss of receptor binding and of biological activity. Thus removal of A21 Asn by caboxypeptidase digestion leads to almost complete loss of biological activity.

Moving to the B-chain, an apparently essential region is the last eight carboxy-terminal amino acids. Many reports exist where the desoctapeptide insulin has been evaluated. In all cases, this molecule shows no biological activity or receptor binding. Whilst B23–30 (Gly-Phe-Phe-Tyr-Thr-Pro-Lys-Thr) appear to be essential for insulin activity the same cannot be said for the residues in the middle of the B-chain. In this case, although there is loss of activity, it is less marked than with modifications in the regions mentioned above. On the whole, it would be fair to say that modification of any of the conserved residues leads to loss of activity. Can this information help us in determining any structure–activity relationships? As with any protein, knowledge of the primary structure alone will not lead to knowledge of how that protein behaves in solution. Knowledge of the tertiary and quaternary structures of insulin is required for a complete analysis of the structural requirements for biological activity.

2.1.2   X-ray analysis and structure–activity relationships

Insulin was first crystallized by Abel in 1926 as rhombohedral crystals (Abel, 1926). The very first X-ray diffraction studies revealed that the molecular mass (M_r) of crystalline insulin was approximately 12 000. Following Sanger's determination of the primary structure of the hormone, showing an M_r of about 6000, it was realized that the M_r derived from the crystallographic studies corresponded to an insulin dimer (Fig. 2.3).

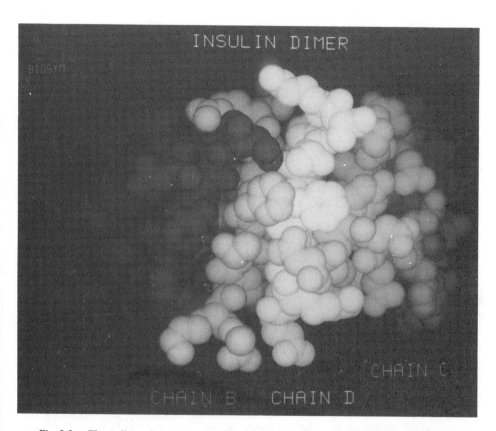

Fig. 2.3 — Three-dimensional structure of insulin. A computer-generated model of the insulin dimer. The figure was produced by Biosym, Inc., under contract from Dr P. W. Jeffs, Head of the Structural and Biophysical Chemistry Department at Glaxo, Inc., who kindly donated it to the author. This illustration is reproduced in colour on the cover of the book.

A complete discussion of the extensive studies on the X-ray analysis of insulin is beyond the scope of this book. The reader is referred in particular to the work of Blundell and colleagues (e.g. Blundell *et al.*, 1972). Here I will present a brief account of the more important inferences from these studies with respect to the biological activity of insulin.

Insulin crystallizes out of aqueous solution in rhombohedral forms containing two to four zinc atoms per six insulin molecules. Each rhombohedral cell (a spherical hexamer) contains three insulin dimers. Each of the two zinc atoms is attached to the insulin moleules through the B10 His residues. Interestingly, the crystal structure of insulin appears to correspond very well with the storage granules present in β-cells. Insulin is stored in sperical hexameric granules containing insulin–zinc crystals. The dimensions of the granules and those of the insulin crystal hexamer are identical: about 50 Å diameter. Insulin appears to retain in physiological solution a structure similar to that of crystalline insulin.

It was pointed out above that certain residues in the primary structure of insulin appear to be of absolute importance in the biological activity of the hormone. In fact, the X-ray studies have revealed a structural domain consisting of the Al Gly, A19–21 (Tyr-Cys-Asn), and the eight carboxy-terminal residues of the B-chain. This region is proposed as the putative receptor-binding domain, and contains the region involved in the formation of insulin dimers. If this is so we would expect the insulin dimer to be the active species and not the monomer. In this context, it is interesting to compare the structures of porcine insulin and that of a hystriocorph such as coypu. The latter is hardly active when compared with the former (less than 10%), and has some regions of obvious difference. Thus, coypu insulin has a sequence of B22–29 Arg-Gly-Phe-Tyr-Arg-Pro-Asn-Asp and no B30 residue; in addition, it has an additional residue of A22 Asp. These differences correspond to the region involved in dimer formation. Hystricomorph insulins do not form dimers, and are poorly active. Blundell and colleagues proposed that the receptor-binding region in the insulin molecule includes the hydrophobic region involved in dimerization and other polar residues close to this area. It is possible, and likely, that other residues and interactions between residues may be important in the binding of insulin to its receptor.

It is difficult to evaluate the physiological or even the therapeutic implications of these studies. In classical pharmacological studies, structure–activity relationships can lead to the production of more potent pharmacophores. In the case of insulin, no other more potent analogue has been produced and, whilst it has been a topic of speculation, the idea of artificial insulins (small organic compounds that would bind insulin receptor) is still a dream.

2.2 INSULIN SYNTHESIS

Regulation of the synthesis of any protein can occur at any of the steps involved. Thus, control may be exerted upon the rates of transcription (i.e. mRNA formation from DNA), translation (conversion of the mRNA transcript into protein) or post-translation modifications of the mature protein. In the case of a secreted protein, such as insulin, control may be exterted, in addition, upon the step converting the precursor protein to the mature product, and on the secretory process itself.

Insulin is derived biosynthetically from a precursor, proinsulin, which consists of the A- and B-chains linked together via the C-peptide (see above and Fig. 2.2). However, preproinsulin, rather than proinsulin, is the translated product. Preproinsulin has an additional N-terminal 24 amino acids (located, therefore, adjacent to the

B-chain) which constitute the signal peptide. Signal peptides are commonly found on secreted proteins, as they allow passage of the molecule through endoplasmic reticulum. Cleavage of preproinsulin to proinsulin occurs in the rough endoplasmic reticulum. The fully folded and oxidized proinsulin molecules are transported to the Golgi apparatus where they are packed into secretory granules. During the formation of secretory granules, proinsulin is cleaved to yield insulin and the C-peptide, which are secreted together. Small amounts of proinsulin can be detected in the plasma of most individuals but they have no physiological function.

With the advent of recombinant DNA technology, the study of genes and their expression has become feasible. This section will examine the insulin gene, its features, and most importantly the regulation of its expression. A basic knowledge of the terminology used in molecular biology is assumed.

2.2.1   The insulin gene
The insulin gene was one of the first human genes to be cloned (Bell *et al.*, 1980). The structure of the gene is shown schematically in Fig. 2.4. The gene is 1500 base pairs

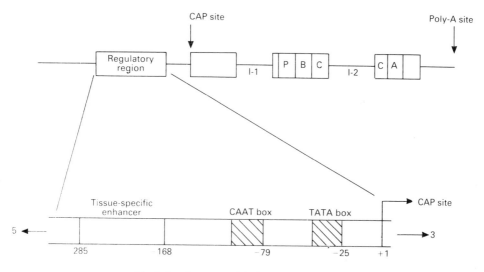

Fig. 2.4 — Structure of the human insulin gene.

(bp) long and contains three exons and two introns (exons are transcribed and present in mature mRNA whereas introns are not). The introns can be of variable length: intron-1 varies from 119 bp in chicken to 179 bp in humans, whereas intron-2 can vary from 264 bp in dog to over 3500 bp in chicken (786 in humans). The location of the introns is highly conserved. Thus, intron-1 is always located adjacent to the untranslated exon-1, while intron-2 always separates the sequences that encode residues 6 and 7 of the C-peptide. Exon-1 begins with the CAP site (where mRNA synthesis begins, and so-called because the 5′ end of the mRNA is said to be capped by the presence of a modified guanine nucleotide) and encodes a region that is transcribed but not translated. Exon-2 contains the sequences encoding the prepeptide, the B-chain and part of the C-peptide. Exon-3 encodes the rest of the C-peptide and the A-chain; it also appears to have an untranslated region following the A-chain.

At either side of the coding sequences, at the so-called 'flanking sequences', the insulin gene contains the two typical features of eukaryotic genes: a transcription promoter (TATAAAG) at the 5′ end, and a polyadenylation site at the 3′ terminus (AATAAA). The transcription promoter, or 'TATA box', is located 24 bp upstream from the CAP site, and, as with all eukaryotic promoters, is required to initiate transcription correctly. The polyadenylation signal resides 20 nucleotides before the polyadenylic acid tail in the mRNA.

Studies on the regulation of gene expression have concentrated mainly on the regulation of transcription. Attention has focused on regions, or sequences, that direct the initiation of transcription, such as promoter elements. These regulatory sequences of eukaryotic genes are found upstream from the CAP site and, in addition to the TATA box mentioned above, include a 'CAAT box', a sequence which in the insulin gene is found 79 bp upstream from the CAP site (Fig. 2.4).

The insulin gene exists as a single copy in most species, except in rats and mice where two copies exist. Interestringly, rat insulin gene I does not have the second intron and exhibits 70% homology to the other copy. In the rat both genes are present in the same chromosome (1) and appear to be transcribed in equal portions. In mice, the genes are in different chromosomes (6 and 7) but this seems to have no effect on the relatively identical rates of transcription. The location of the insulin gene in humans is on band p15 of the short arm of chromosome 11.

In addition to the features described above, the human insulin gene has some characteristics that make it different from that of other species. The structure of the flanking sequences at both ends of the message is unusual. At about 6000 bp downstream and 15 000 bp upstream, there are repetitive sequences considered to be members of the so-called 'Alu family'. The Alu family are repetitive regions of 300 bp found distributed across the whole genome whose function is totally unknown. The name derives from the observation that these repetitive sequences contain a cleavage site recognized by the restriction endonuclease AluI. The sequences at the 3′ end are not polymorphic, whereas those at the 5′ end are polymorphic, consisting of varying numbers of repeats with a consensus sequence ACAGGGGTGTGGGG. These regions have been implicated in the incidence of both diabetes and atherosclerosis, but this suggestion remains controversial (see for instance, Mandrup-Poulsen et al., 1985).

2.2.2 Regulation of insulin gene expression

The regulation of the expression of eukaryotic genes is an area still in the early stages of inception and advance. Many of the recent developments in molecular biology have provided the tools to reach an understanding of how genes can be switched on or off. As indicated above, most of the recent research in this area has focused on the regulation of transcription, with the emphasis being on the upstream sequences believed to contain the 'promoter elements'. These sequences can interact with proteins that can thereby affect the reading of the DNA message. In addition to the TATA box and the CAAT box, both of which are found on the insulin gene, there are 'glucocorticoid-responsive elements'. No evidence for the latter has been found on the insulin gene.

A method that has become standard in the study of the function of promoters is the introduction of cloned promoter sequences into mammalian genes by any of the several techniques available (see any molecular biology textbook for details of these techniques). Typically, the promoter sequence is ligated to a gene coding for an enzyme that can be easily assayed, e.g. the bacterial chloramphenicol acetyltransferase (CAT). This 'reporter gene' is then introduced into the cells of interest. This approach has been used in the study of the regulation of the expression of the insulin gene by its promoters. Introduction of 'reporter genes' containing the insulin promoter sequence into pancreatic and non-pancreatic cells has identified regions that are required for tissue-specific gene expression. The work of Rutter and his colleagues has shown that expression of the insulin gene can occur only in pancreatic cells†. Using a reporter gene consisting of the insulin gene promoter and CAT, they found sequences that directed the tissue specificity. Furthermore, the region responsible for this regulation was narrowed down to 90 bp residing between −168 and −258 bp from the CAP site (see Fig. 2.4) (Walker et al., 1983; Nir et al., 1986). This region of 90 bp appears to enhance the tissue-specific transcription of any gene even if moved many base pairs further away. It is thus referred to as an 'enhancer', i.e. a region capable of stimulating transcription in both orientations and of acting at a distance.

Thus, in summary, 5′ flanking sequences of the insulin gene determine the tissue-specific expression of the gene. This conclusion has also been confirmed in transgenic mice (Hanahan, 1985). Two control elements, an enhancer and a promoter, are involved in the pancreatic cell-specific regulation. In order to clarify this somewhat complex system, Edlund, Rutter and colleagues have carried out a series of studies using mutational analysis of the promoter region. The mutational analysis is done by assembling a series of overlapping oligonucleotides of 20 bp in length in such a way that short sequences of base pairs can be altered without changing the length of the elements (Karlsson et al., 1987). These studies identified two short repeating sequences centred at −108 and at −237 in the 5′ flanking region that appear to play a critical role. In a more recent follow-up study, Rutter and colleagues have shown that the glucose-responsive transcriptional elements reside in these two regions (from −104 to −112 and from −233 to −241) (Moss et al., 1988).

In addition to these regulatory systems, the insulin gene promoter may contain a region that binds to a repressor protein (Nir et al., 1986), and thus enables negative regulation of transcription. The binding of a repressor protein may prevent the binding of a positive regulator or place the DNA in such a conformation that it becomes unstable. The repressor proteins could also exist in non-pancreatic tissues, thereby further ensuring tissue-specific expression of the insulin gene.

Whilst the discussion above may explain some of the molecular mechanisms regulating insulin gene expression, the means whereby this is achieved physiologically, *in vivo*, have not been referred to, and are clearly of importance in the maintainance of normal glycaemic control.

---

† This observation is of importance since the insulin mRNA has been located in other cell types such as neurons by *in situ* hybridization (see for instance Schechter et al., 1988). It is possible and likely that in these cells insulin is not expressed and secreted as it is in pancreas.

2.2.3   Physiological regulation of gene expression

The coordinated physiological regulation of the processes whereby normal glucose levels are maintained must involve regulation of insulin synthesis — and hence of gene expression — by similar mechanisms, or compounds, to those that regulate the secretion of insulin. The assumption behind this statement is obviously that the processes of secretion and synthesis are complementary. A basic observation in support of this conclusion is that the total insulin content of the pancreas decreases only slightly after many hours of infusion of glucose. Therefore the insulin that is being secreted is being replaced by newly synthesized insulin. Consequently, it is fair to make the assumption that, on the whole, the biosynthetic process for insulin reflects or represents accurately and directly the expression of its gene. Whilst this may not necessarily be so, the generalization appears to obtain.

It has long been known that glucose stimulates the incorporation of labelled leucine into insulin (Howell & Taylor, 1966). This is taken to indicate clearly that glucose stimulates insulin biosynthesis as well as secretion. In more recent times, glucose has been shown by several laboratories to stimulate the expression of the insulin gene itself, in islets from both rodents and humans (Welsh *et al.*, 1985; Giddings *et al.*, 1985; Hammonds *et al.*, 1987a,b) (see below for further details). Thus, glucose exerts potent regulatory control at transcriptional and translational levels. It is interesting, in fact, to compare the dose–response curves of glucose's effects on insulin biosynthesis and secretion. Biosynthesis appears to be more sensitive to changes in glucose concentrations. Thus, the half-maximal effects occur at approximately 3 mM for synthesis and over 6 mM for secretion. The effect of glucose on insulin biosynthesis is rapid and maintained for a long period, suggesting that enough insulin is stored to ensure an adequate response upon a subsequent challenge.

All compounds that stimulate insulin secretion also appear to stimulate insulin biosynthesis (see for instance Table 1 in Campbell *et al.*, 1982), with the notable exception of the sulphonylureas, which enhance glucose-stimulated insulin release. Overall, it is therefore fair to say that the processes of biosynthesis and secretion are closely interrelated, if not dependent on each other. But what of gene expression itself?

Instead of examining biosynthetic rates, it is possible to measure the actual content of preproinsulin mRNA. Moreover, this measurement will actually show if the biosynthetic rates do reflect accurately the rate of gene epxression. Two methods exist for measuring the amount of mRNA: a cell-free translation assay of RNA isolated from islets, and a hybridization assay using a radiolabelled recombinant cDNA probe, a method which is highly sensitive. Not many studies of this type exist, but those that do come to the same conclusion. Glucose does indeed regulate insulin biosynthesis at both translational and transcriptional levels, but there is a time shift in these effects. Thus, transcriptional effects are long-term, whereas the translational effects occur in the short term. Some evidence to support this conclusion is that the glucose-stimulated increase in the amount of preproinsulin mRNA is not observed until two hours after glucose administration, and is then maintained for about 24 hours. On the other hand, after one hour there is an increase in insulin biosynthesis without a change in mRNA levels (see e.g. Itoh & Okamoto, 1980). When the time course of these events is compared to that of glucose stimulation of insulin secretion, it is clear that the immediate response of the islets is secretory, with the effect on the expression of the gene restoring the depleted granules.

In contrast to experiments in rodent islets, fewer studies have been done using human islets. Glucose also stimulates preproinsulin mRNA levels as well as secretion in these islets (Hammonds et al., 1987b). The shift in the time frame for these effects is also the same as in rodents. In a comprehensive study, Hammonds and colleagues showed that the effects of glucose on preproinsulin mRNA levels occurred in two phases: an initial short-term phase involving post-transcriptional control, and a long-term regulation under transcriptional control. Moreover, they presented evidence for the possibility that a peptide (perhaps insulin itself!) may regulate the levels of the mRNA. This suggests the ability of insulin to feedback on its own synthesis. Their work also showed that important differences exist between rodents and humans where the effects of protein kinase C activators are concerned. Although phorbol esters (which activate protein kinase C) cause a potentiation of insulin secretion both in rodents and humans, they inhibit preproinsulin mRNA accumulation in human islets. The observation that various agonists can modulate the expression of the insulin gene may be of potential therapeutic importance if pathological defects are shown to occur on the expression of the gene.

2.2.4   Pathology of insulin gene expression
The clinical importance of any physiological system becomes obvious when the system is shown to be solely or particularly responsible for a disease process. Few good animal models of type II diabetes exist, but in one of them a defective insulin gene expression can be shown to correlate with the dvelopment of diabetes. Streptozotocin-treated newborn rats develop a syndrome similar to type II diabetes as they become adults. When they reach four weeks of age the animals are glucose-intolerant and show a 50% fall in the rate of insulin biosynthesis and in the levels of mRNA (Permutt et al., 1984). To date, no studies exist on the expression of the insulin gene in type II diabetic patients.

2.3   INSULIN SECRETION
The secretion of insulin by the pancreatic β-cells is the most important factor in the regulation of glucose homeostasis. Absence of or decrease in this ability will result in diabetes. These two statements may, by now, seem obvious, but it is worth stressing that an increased rate of secretion of insulin is an absolute requirement for the body to decrease a rapid elevation in plasma glucose. The process of insulin secretion is a classic example of 'stimulus–secretion coupling'. This could make the process interesting in its own right, but the manifest clinical importance of the coupling between high plasma glucose concentration and the release of insulin requires, and deserves, close examination and understanding.

The most important physiological regulator of insulin secretion is glucose. The pancreas is exquisitely sensitive to changes in glucose concentrations. Although other nutrients also cause the release of insulin, glucose is the only substrate that can do so at physiological concentrations. Many other regulators exist, including other nutrients, hormones, and neurotransmitters.

Although the stimulus–response coupling for insulin has been studied in considerable detail for many years, the complexities of this system have not decreased (!). To date, all of the well-characterized systems of signal transduction (cAMP, Ca^{2+}, IP_3/protein kinase C) appear to be involved in regulating the secretion of insulin.

The mechanisms by which glucose and other secretagogues cause the release of insulin from the pancreas have been studied extensively since methods for the isolation of islets of Langerhans became known and established (see, for instance, Hellerstrom, 1964; Moskalewski, 1965; Keen et al., 1965). These methods allowed the making of the basic observations that have led to our current concept of the regulation of insulin secretion. Thus, the discovery of a relationship between glucose metabolism and insulin secretion (Randle et al., 1968) and of the requirement for extracellular Ca^{2+} (Grodsky & Bennett, 1966) are but two of a long list of early studies.

In this section, I will review the mechanisms involved in the coupling between plasma glucose and insulin secretion and the role of the Ca^{2+}, cAMP and phosphoinositide messenger systems in hormone release. Many reviews exist, and this section is, in essence, a review of reviews. The reader is referred specially to the reviews by Ashcroft (1980), Howell (1984), Turk et al. (1987) and Prentki and Matschinski (1987).

2.3.1 Morphology of the islets of Langerhans

The islets of Langerhans are composed of four different types of cells. The A- or α-cells secrete glucagon and constitute 20% of all cell types. The B- or β-cells secrete insulin and represent about 75% of the islet. The two other less well known types are the somatostatin-containing D- or δ-cells representing about 3–5% of all cells and the F-cells which secrete the pancreatic polypeptide and constitute under 2% of the islet (Table 2.1). Within the islet, the β-cells form its medulla; that is, they congregate in

Table 2.1 — Cell type and secretory products in the islets of Langerhans

Cell type	Percentage of Islet cell mass	Secretory product
A (α)	20	Glucagon, proglucagon
B (β)	75	Insulin, C-peptide, proinsulin
D (δ)	3–5	Somatostatin
F (PP)	<2	Pancreatic polypeptide

the centre of the islet. The cortex seems to contain contiguous α-, β-, and δ-cells and often appears to invaginate the islet along the blood vessel (Fig. 2.5).

The close proximity of those cell types has suggested the possibility of cell–cell interactions and of paracrine regulation of their secretory products. Thus it is known that glucagon stimulates insulin secretion from the β-cells (through a cAMP-mediated mechanism) and of somatostatin from the δ-cells. On the other hand, somatostatin inhibits the secretion of both glucagon and insulin, whilst insulin exerts

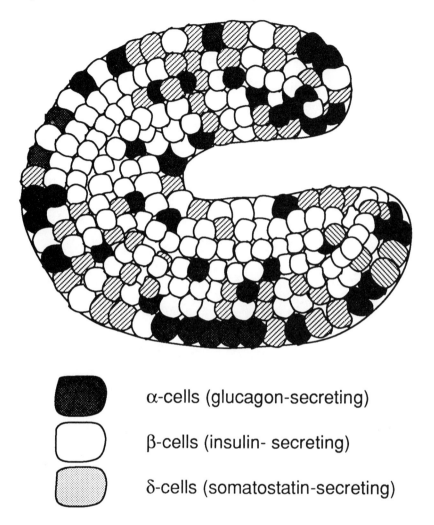

α-cells (glucagon-secreting)

β-cells (insulin- secreting)

δ-cells (somatostatin-secreting)

Fig. 2.5 — Cell types across the islet. (Adapted from Unger (1985).)

inhibition of glucagon alone. It must be emphasized that these relationships have been examined in *in vitro* studies. It is therefore difficult to determine whether in the normal physiological situation, or even in pathological conditions, paracrine control exists, or if regulation of secretion of insulin or glucagon is exerted by substrates or other hormones. The roles of glucagon and somatostatin are beyond the scope of this book and the reader is referred to Unger (1985) and Reichlin (1983) respectively for reviews on these topics.

2.3.1.1 *Insulin storage in the islet*
As was mentioned above (section 2.1.2), insulin is stored in spherical hexameric granules containing insulin–zinc crystals. The insulin storage granule is smaller than

the insulin crystals that can be grown *in vitro*, but its size (0.2–0.3 μm) is similar to that of other hormone storage granules. In addition to insulin, the storage granule contains C-peptide in equimolar amounts, thereby explaining the observed co-secretion of C-peptide with insulin. Calcium, biogenic amines, and enzymes such as acid phosphatase, Ca^{2+}/Mg^{2+}-dependent ATPases and proinsulin-converting enzymes are all also present in the storage granule. The role of the these components of the granule is not clear at all, even though their presence is well-documented.

The presence of Ca^{2+} is particularly strange. The insulin storage granule is estimated to contain somewhere in the region of 100 mM Ca^{2+}. This extraordinary high Ca^{2+} content must imply that there are Ca^{2+}-accumulating mechanisms operating in the granule membrane. Interestingly, the Ca^{2+} content of the granule cannot be decreased even by incubating granules in high Na^+ concentrations. Therefore, once granules have taken up Ca^{2+} they are impermeable to it. It has been suggested that Ca^{2+} and Zn^{2+} both enter the granules in a bound form by mechanisms transporting insulin, other proteins or adenine nucleotides. Thus, all the Ca^{2+} is bound and cannot be released because the permeability of the granules to divalent ions certainly is very low (see Prentki & Matschinski, 1987, for discussion).

The small size of the granules requires there to be large numbers of them in the β-cell in order to store the known content of insulin. In an interesting calculation, Howell (1984) suggests a total of approximately 1.3×10^{13} granules per pancreas. Assuming that 5% of the insulin is secreted per hour, he works out that around 200 million granules are exocytosed per second! As he describes it: 'a rather frequent event'! The insulin storage granules are thus released at a very high rate. It is unclear if the granule is a passive agent or an active participant in the process of exocytosis. One of the possible ways in which active participation could be achieved would be if the granule contained myosin. The granule could thus contribute to its secretion by interacting with the cytoskeleton, which has been implicated in the process of secretion.

2.3.1.2 The islet cytoskeleton

The involvement of microtubules and microfilaments in the process of insulin secretion has been suggested by many experiments. Perhaps the first observations were those of Lacy *et al.* (1968) who showed that colchicine, an agent causing microtubule polymerization, inhibited insulin secretion. Agents that inhibit poly-merization and those that cause depolymerization both result in inhibition of insulin secretion. Study has concentrated on the role of phosphorylation of microtubular proteins. Thus, polymerization of tubulin is increased by increases in the concentra-tion of cAMP. Furthermore, Ca^{2+}–calmodulin-dependent protein kinase (hereafter referred to as Ca/CM-K) can cause the phosphorylation and polymerization of tubulin.

A similar system may operate in the regulation of microfilament assembly; namely, protein phosphorylation may extert a role in this process. In the islet, less than 50% of actin is present in the polymerized form (or F-form). The degree of polymerization is enhanced in parallel with increases in insulin secretion. Thus, polymerization of actin and insulin secretion occur concomitantly. It follows from this relationship that regulation of polymerization of actin will play a role in the secretory process.

The regulation of actin polymerization appears to involve various actin-binding proteins, such as gelsolin, synexin, actinogelin, caldesmon, etc. These proteins bind to non-polymerized actin (or G-actin) and prevent it from polymerizing. Interestingly, a large number of these proteins bind Ca^{2+} and therefore when intracellular Ca^{2+} levels are elevated the actin-binding proteins lose their tight binding onto actin, which is now able to polymerize. The actual details of this system are unclear, as is the possible involvement of actinomyosin in granule movement (in analogy with the muscular system). Myosin and myosin chain kinase have been found in islets but their direct involvement in the secretory system is unclear. Phosphorylated myosin could associate with polymerized actin and thus elicit the contraction of microfilaments. The regulation of myosin chain kinase appears to involve Ca^{2+}/calmodulin and hence a link exists between all the above processes (Fig. 2.6).

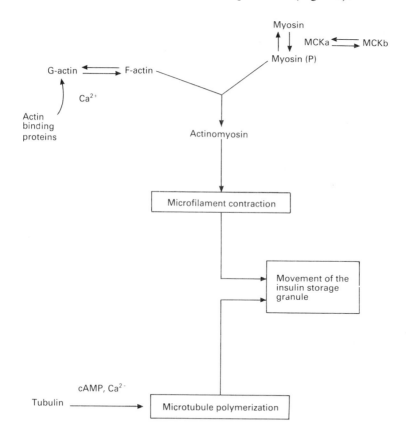

Fig. 2.6 — Involvement of the cytoskeleton in insulin secretion. MCKa and MCKb denote the active and inactive forms of myosin chain kinase respectively. See text for details.

The need for the involvement of the cytoskeleton in insulin secretion is also shown by electron microscopic studies that show the association of secretory granules with microtubules and the direction of them towards the plasma membrane.

Other microscopic studies using video cameras to record the actual movement of granules, show that the process is calcium-dependent. It is also clear from the discussion above that Ca^{2+} is a key regulator of the processes of microtubule polymerization and microfilament contraction. The mechanisms by which Ca^{2+} may do this and the role of Ca^{2+} in the secretory process in general are discussed in detail in section 2.3.3.

2.3.2   Glucose metabolism in the β-cell

Glucose is clearly the most important secretagogue of insulin. The mechanisms by which glucose causes the release of insulin from the pancreas have been the topic of many papers and reviews. By far the clearest exposition of this is in Ashcroft's 1980 review. In this section, I present an overview of his work.

How does the pancreatic β-cell recognize glucose? Two hypotheses have been proposed, both of which are referred to as the 'glucoreceptor model'. In the first such model glucose binds to a membrane protein — a classical 'receptor' — which transmits this signal intracellularly to the various pathways involved in insulin secretion. This model was one of the first suggestions in the attempts to clarify the recognition of glucose. Unfortunately for the hypothesis no such receptor protein has ever been identified. Furthermore, the evidence accrued supports the second alternative. In this model, the 'glucoreceptor' is the metabolism of glucose itself (and hence, perhaps, one enzyme acts as the 'receptor'). It is hypothesized that in the breakdown of glucose one or more intermediates are generated that link glucose breakdown with the process of secretion, thereby acting as triggers. Clearly, the hypothesis could be invalidated if the metabolism of glucose and the secretion of insulin could be separated by some experimental technique, such as the use of metabolic inhibitors. In all the studies performed to date no such inhibition has been shown.

Ashcroft and colleagues have examined over the years many sugars and derivatives for their effects on secretion of insulin (see Ashcroft, 1980). The first interesting observation is that only glucose, mannose and N-acetylglucosamine cause stimulation of insulin release and of biosynthesis, and are also metabolized by the islets. Non-metabolizable sugars such as 3-O-methylglucose or 2-deoxyglucose do not cause secretion or synthesis of insulin. In addition, substrates that may enter glycolysis at a lower point in the pathway, such as glyceraldehyde or dihydroxyacetone, also cause secretion and synthesis (Fig. 2.7). As a general rule, there is also good agreement between the rates of metabolism of the sugar and the rates of secretion or biosynthesis of the hormone.

The use of inhibitors of glycolysis has been very useful in the identification of the key regulatory step linking metabolism and secretion. Thus, mannoheptulose inhibits glucokinase and causes inhibition of insulin release by glucose and mannose, but not by N-acetylglucosamine. Iodoacetate, which inhibits further down the glycolytic pathway inhibits the stimulation of secretion by all sugars. These and other data have led Ashcroft and colleagues (and indeed other authors) to suggest that the 'glucoreceptor' is the phosphorylation of glucose, a reaction which, in the islets, is catalysed by glucokinase.

Glucokinase differs from hexokinase in its K_m for glucose; the values are 10–20 mM and 0.1 mM respectively. It is worth stating the obvious advantage for the

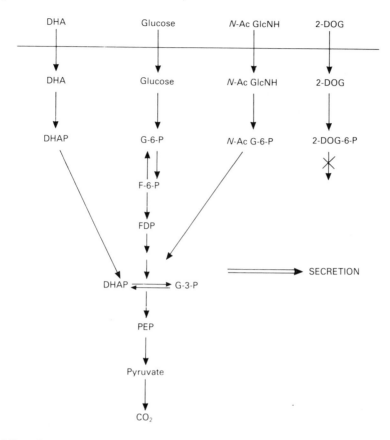

Fig. 2.7 — Sugar metabolism in the β-cell. DHA: Dihydroxyacetone; N-Ac GlcNH: N-acetylgluco-samine; 2-DOG: 2-deoxyglucose; G-6-P: glucose-6-phosphate; F-6-P: fructose-6-phosphate; FDP: fructose-1,6-diphosphate; DHAP: dihydroxyacetone phosphate; PEP: phosphoeuolypyruvate.

islet in having glucokinase and not hexokinase. If the β-cells responded to glucose concentrations as low as 0.1 mM — as they would if they possessed hexokinase — the cirulating plasma concentration of glucose would cause constant maximal stimulation of insulin release and hypoglycaemia would ensue. On the other hand, glucokinase will only become catalytically effective at concentrations of glucose above physiological levels and hence only lead to insulin release when the plasma glucose concentration is elevated, e.g. following a meal. Islets are similar to the liver in this respect, and also in possessing glucose-6-phosphatase. However, the relative contribution of this enzyme to the overall glucose utilization rate is unknown.

In summary, glucose metabolism is necessary to elicit insulin secretion, and the key step in this pathway in the β-cell — the 'glucoreceptor' — is probably glucokinase. Does glucose metabolism interact with other mechanisms involved in the secretory process, and if so how? Firstly, let us consider the main molecular mechanisms leading to the secretion of insulin.

2.3.3 Role of Ca^{2+} in insulin secretion
It has been well established that insulin secretion is absolutely dependent on extracellular Ca^{2+}. Many studies suggest that elevation of cytosolic Ca^{2+} is necessary

for secretion and that biphasic changes in Ca^{2+} concentration may explain in part the biphasic nature of glucose stimulation of insulin release (Fig. 2.8). Therefore, Ca^{2+}

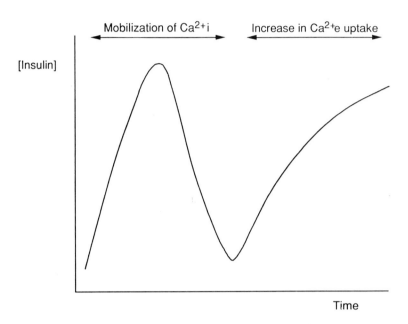

$$Ca^{2+}i = \text{Intracellular } Ca^{2+}; \quad Ca^{2+}e = \text{extracellular } Ca^{2+}$$

Fig. 2.8 — Phases of glucose-induced insulin release. $Ca^{2+}i$, intracellular Ca^{2+}; $Ca^{2+}e$, extracellular Ca^{2+}.

appears as the most important second messenger in stimulus–secretion coupling. The role of Ca^{2+} in insulin secretion is a topic that has been extensively studied and reviewed in considerable detail. This information is well beyond the scope of this book and I therefore recommend to the reader the reviews by Wollheim & Sharp (1981) and, more recently, Prentki & Matschinski (1987). I will summarize briefly the current hypotheses.

Glucose enhances Ca^{2+} uptake from the extracellular medium, and so do other secretagogues such as mannose or glyceraldehyde, as well as the sulphonylureas. Glucose also causes a transient decrease in Ca^{2+} efflux. The use of Ca^{2+} channel inhibitors, such a verapamil, has suggested that the first, rapid, phase of glucose-induced insulin secretion may be dependent upon the mobilization of intracellular stores of Ca^{2+}, wheras the second phase is due to glucose-induced stimulation of Ca^{2+} uptake from extracellular sources (Fig. 2.8) (see Wollheim & Sharp, 1981 or Hedeskov, 1980).

Glucose causes depolarization of the β-cell membrane which leads to the opening of a voltage-sensitive Ca^{2+} channel. This process appears to be due, in turn, to the closure of a K^+ channel. Glucose and other secretagogues have been shown to cause the closure of the K^+ channel (Ashcroft *et al.*, 1984; Cook & Hales, 1984; Misler *et al.*, 1986). The glucose-sensitive K^+ channel has also been shown to be closed by ATP (Misler *et al.*, 1986) and therefore changes in the ATD/ADP ratio, as would occur during glycolysis, may regulate the activity of the channel. It is of course possible that many other systems regulate the activity of the K^+ channel, such as cAMP, the phosphoinositides, protein kinase C, etc., but whilst the idea may be attractive in terms of integration of regulatory pathways, the evidence at present is highly preliminary (see Prentki & Matschinski (1987) for a full account). Recently, the sulphonylurea receptor has been identified as the ATP-sensitive K^+ channel (see Boyd, 1988) and this may explain some of the characteristics of the effects of sulphonylureas on insulin secretion.

Neurotransmitters and other agonists cause an increase in cytosolic Ca^{2+} concentration by the inositol trisphosphate (IP_3)-mediated mobilization of Ca^{2+} from the endoplasmic reticulum. Agonist binding to its receptor induces the activation of a phospholipase C resulting in the generation of diacylglycerol (DG) and IP_3. The latter causes elevation of cytosolic Ca^{2+}, while DG activities protein kinase C (details of this second-messenger system will be found in Chapter 6). Interestingly, glucose appears to cause the breakdown of phosphatidylinositol polyphosphates in a Ca^{2+}-dependent manner. Prentki & Matschinski (1987) suggest that glucose stimulation of inositol lipid breakdown would result in DAG activation of protein kinase C, which may be involved in the second phase of insulin release, and in IP_3-mediated elevation of cytosolic Ca^{2+}, thereby maintaining an elevated Ca^{2+} concentration.

The elevated intracellular Ca^{2+} concentration leads to the activation of a variety of Ca^{2+}-sensitive or -dependent proteins, such as Ca^{2+}/CM-K and protein kinase C. These can then promote the phosphorylation of target proteins that may be involved in movement of the insulin storage granules (see Turk *et al.*, 1987). A summary of the involvement of Ca^{2+} is presented in Fig. 2.9.

2.3.4   Role of cAMP in insulin secretion
Various agonists that induce secretion do so by increasing the intracellular concentration of cAMP. The effects of all these agonists (glucagon, forskolin, etc.) are only seen however at high glucose concentrations. Thus, they do not stimulate insulin release in the absence of glucose. Moreover, glucose has been reported to cause a small increase in the concentration of cAMP in the islet (Charles *et al.*, 1975).

The mechanism of stimulation of insulin secretion by cAMP is mediated through protein phosphorylation. Many papers have reported changes in the phosphorylation state of several islet proteins in response to changes in the cAMP concentration. Little is known about the identity or role of any of these proteins, as they are characterized by their relative molecular masses on polyacrylamide gels. Undoubtedly, the cytoskeletal proteins have been implicated (see above).

cAMP could also have effects other than phosphorylation of cytoskeletal proteins. It is possible that it may cause the phosphorylation and activation of Ca^{2+} channels or the inactivation of the K^+ channel (see the review by Rasmussen & Barrett (1984) for discussion of this topic). In addition, the cAMP and the IP_3/DG second-messenger systems are known to interact with each other, in many cell types, and thus modulate the response of the Ca^{2+} system, thereby regulating the sensitivity of the β-cell to different stimuli.

Two second-messenger systems (cAMP and IP_3/DG), Ca^{2+} uptake and glucose

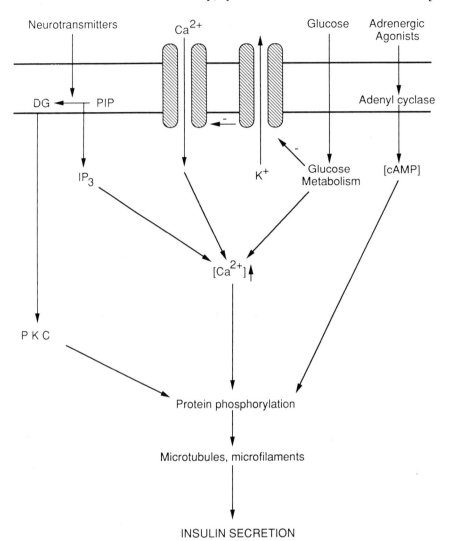

Fig. 2.9 — Pathways involved in insulin secretion. DG: Diacylglycerol; IP$_3$: Inostol, 1,4,5 tris
phosphate; PIP$_2$: Phosphatidylinosital 4,5 bis phosphate; PKC: Protein Kinase C.

metabolism, become integrated in the regulation of insulin secretion (Fig. 2.9). Yet,
in spite of all the detailed knowledge concerning these molecular mechanisms, two
major questions remain unanswered. Firstly, what causes the biphasic nature of
insulin release and secondly, what are the mechanisms involved in the desensitization of the β-cell to glucose, as observed in type II diabetes? These critical issues
remain unresolved.

REFERENCES

Abel, J. J. (1926) *Proc. Natl. Acad. Sci. USA* **12**, 12–136.
Ashcroft, S. J. H. (1980) *Diabetologia* **18**, 5–15.

Ashcroft, F. M., Harrison, D. E. & Ashcroft, S. J. H. (1984) *Nature* **312**, 446–448.

Bell, G. I., Pictet, R. L., Rutter, W. J., Cordell, B., Tischer, E. & Goodman, H. M. (1980) *Nature* **284**, 26–32.

Blundell, T. L., Dodson, G. G., Hodgkin, D. C. & Mercola, D. A. (1972) *Adv. Protein Chem.* **26**, 279.

Boyd, A. E. (1988) *Diabetes* **37**, 847–851.

Campbell, I. L., Hellquist, N. B. & Taylor, K. W. (1982) *Clin. Sci.* **62**, 449–455.

Charles, M. A., Lawecki, J., Pictet, R. & Grodski, G. M. (1975) *J. Biol. Chem.* **250**, 6134–6140.

Cook, D. L. & Hales, C. N. (1984) *Nature* **311**, 271–273.

Giddings, S. J., Chirgwing, J. M. & Permutt, M. A. (1985) *Diabetes Res.* **2**, 71–75.

Grodski, G. M. & Bennett, L. L. (1966) *Diabetes* **15**, 910–913.

Hanahan, D. (1985) *Nature* **315**, 115–122.

Hammonds, P., Schofield, P. N. & Ashcroft, S. J. H. (1987a) *FEBS Lett.* **213**, 149–154.

Hammonds, P., Schofield, P. N., Ashcroft, S. J. H., Sutton, R. & Gray, D. W. R. (1987b) *FEBS Lett.* **223**, 131–137.

Hedeskov, C. (1980) *Physiol. Rev.* **60**, 442–509.

Hellerstrom, C. (1964) *Acta Endocrinol.* **45**, 122–132.

Howell, S. L. (1984) *Diabetologia* **26**, 319–327.

Howell, S. L. & Taylor, K. W. (1966) *Biochim. Biophys. Acta* **130**, 519–521.

Itoh, N. & Okamoto, H. (1980) *Nature* **283**, 100–102.

Karlsson, O., Edlund, T., Moss, J. B., Rutter, W. J. & Walker, M. D. (1987) *Proc. Natl. Acad. Sci. USA* **84**, 8819–8823.

Keen, H., Sells, R. & Jarret, R. J. (1965) *Diabetologia* **1**, 28–32.

Lacy, P. E., Howell, S. L., Young, D. A. & Fink, C. J. (1968) *Nature* **219**, 1177–1179.

Mandrup-Poulsen, T., Owerbach, D., Nerup, J., Johansen, K., Ingerslov, J. & Tybjaerg-Hansen, A. (1985) *Diabetologia* **28**, 556–564.

Misler, S., Falke, L. C., Gillis, K. & McDaniel, M. L. (1986) *Proc. Natl. Acad. Sci. USA* **83**, 7119–7123.

Moskalewski, S. (1965) *Gen. Com. Endocrinol.* **5**, 342–353.

Moss, L. G., German, M. S. & Rutter, W. J. (1988) *Diabetes* **37**, Suppl. 1, 48A (Abstract No. 192).

Nir, U., Walker, M. D. & Rutter, W. J. (1986) *Proc. Natl. Acad. Sci. USA* **83**, 3180–3184.

Permutt, M. A., Kakita, K., Malinas, P., Karl, I., Bonnerweir, S., Weir, G. & Giddings, S. J. (1984) *J. Clin. Invest.* **73**, 1344–1350.

Prentki, M. & Matschinski, F. M. (1987) *Physiol. Rev.* **67**, 1185–1248.

Rasmussen, H. & Barrett, P. Q. (1984) *Physiol. Rev.* **64**, 938–984.

Randle, P. J., Ascroft, S. J. H. & Gill, J. R. (1968) In *Carbohydrate metabolism*, Dickens, F., Randle, P. J. & Wheelan, W. J. (Eds) Vol. 1, Academic Press, London, pp. 427–447.

Reichlin, S. (1983) *N. Eng. J. Med.* **309**, 1495.

Ryle, A. P., Sanger, F., Smith, L. F. & Kitoi, R. (1955) *Biochem. J.* **60**, 541–566.

Schechter, R., Holtzclaw, L., Sadiq, F., Kahn, A. & Devaskar, S. (1988) *Endocrinology* **123**, 505–513.

Turk, J., Wolk, B. A. & McDaniel, M. L. (1987) *Prog. Lipid Res.* **26**, 125–181.
Unger, R. H. (1985) *Diabetologia* **28**, 574.
Walker, M. D., Edlund, T., Boulet, A. M. & Rutter, W. J. (1983) *Nature* **306**, 557–561.
Welsh, M., Nielsen, D. A., Mackrell, A. J. & Steiner, D. F. (1985) *J. Biol. Chem.* **260**, 13 590–13 595.
Wollheim, C. B. & Sharp, G. W. G. (1981) *Physiol. Rev.* **61**, 914–973.

3

Pathophysiology of insulin

3.1 INTRODUCTION

Diabetes and its complications is one of the leading causes of death in Europe and in the United States. The disease affects up to 3% of the population of Britain and up to 5% of Americans. Although the acute, short-term effects of diabetes may be controlled by administation of insulin, the long-term complications of the disease are often fatal. Diabetes is the main cause of blindness in Britain and other countries, and diabetics have an extraordinarily high incidence of renal failure (up to 17 times higher than the rest of the population), cardiovascular disease, and gangrene.

Diabetes has been recognized for about 2000 years, but treatment only became available following the discovery of insulin (see Chapter 1). It is important however to realize what disease one is referring to. Diabetes is classified into two types, often described as juvenile onset and maturity onset, also known as type I and type II respectively. A more clinical definition, and one which accurately describes the major feature of the disease, is the classification of diabetics into insulin-dependent (or IDDM) and non-insulin-dependent (or NIDDM). A discussion of the clinical profile and the physiological processes involved in the two types of diabetes is presented in this chapter. Prior to this, it is necessary to discuss the physiological roles of insulin so that we may understand the pathology of diabetic patients.

3.2 METABOLIC EFFECTS OF INSULIN

3.2.1 Effects on carbohydrate metabolism

The effects of insulin on muscle and adipose tissue are discussed together because in these tissues the direct effects of insulin are similar and occur by the same or similar mechanisms. Both are glucose utilizing tissues, where insulin stimulates glucose breakdown and glycogen synthesis. The liver however is a gluconeogenic tissue and insulin's effects here are more complex than in the other tissues.

3.2.1.1 Muscle and adipose tissue
3.2.1.1.1 Glucose utilization

Insulin increases the rate of glucose metabolism in skeletal muscle and this can be accounted for by effects on glucose transport, glycolysis and glycogen synthesis.

The insulin stimulation of glucose transport across the cell membrane is due to an increase in the V_{max} of the process with little, if any, effect on the K_m. The increase in V_{max} is thought to be the result of an increase in the number of functional carrier molecules in the cell membrane. The mechanism of translocation of glucose transporter molecules to the cell membrane is described in detail in section 4.3.2.

The increase in glucose transport results in an increase in the rate of glycolysis, probably by internal communication through the pathway (Fig. 3.1). The increase in intracellular concentration of glucose will lead to an increase in the rate of its phosphorylation by hexokinase and hence ultimately in the overall glycolytic flux. No significant increases in the activities of any of the glycolytic enzymes have been shown with insulin.†

An increased glycolytic rate will lead to an increase in pyruvate concentration and thus in the rate of glucose oxidation. The reaction catalysed by pyruvate dehydrogenase commits pyruvate to oxidation to acetyl CoA and is therefore a point of no return for the glucose carbon, since acetyl CoA cannot be converted back to glucose. In muscle this reaction leads to production of CO_2 and supply of energy. In liver and adipose tissue, on the other hand, this acetyl CoA can be used for the synthesis of lipids. Regulation of this enzyme is thus of major importance for the control of overall glucose metabolism.

In man, the oxidation of glucose is increased by exercise and decreased by diabetes, starvation, high-fat diets and oxidation of lipids. In animal models, the activity of pyruvate dehydrogenase is correlated with the rate of glucose oxidation when this is altered by the conditions mentioned above. This form of regulation provides the molecular basis for a reciprocal (as opposed to dependent) interrelationship between glucose and fat. This relationship forms the basis of the hypothesis of the glucose/fatty acid cycle, originally formulated by Randle and his colleagues in 1963. It is important to dwell temporarily on this topic as it provides the basis of understanding the physiological role of insulin.

The basic proposal of the glucose/fatty acid cycle is that in conditions when carbohydrate stores are low (e.g. when glycogen stores in the liver or muscle are depleted, for instance, following exercise), fatty acids are mobilized from adipose tissue so that they may be oxidized by skeletal muscle. This, in turn, inhibits glucose oxidation by muscle. Conversely, when carbohydrates are replenished the rate of lipolysis in adipose tissue decreases (as re-esterification of the fatty acids to triglycerides occurs) and hence the rate of glucose utilization by muscle now increases (Fig. 3.2). The underlying mechanism of glucose inhibition is an increase in

---

† It is important to refer the reader to textbooks on metabolic regulation. The author's preferences are E. A. Newsholme's two books, both of which are referenced at the end.

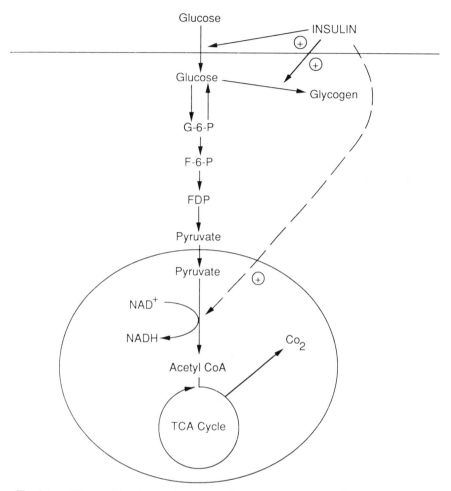

Fig. 3.1 — Effects of insulin on glucose metabolism in muscle and adipose tissue. Insulin stimulates glucose transport across the membrane and has direct effects on glycogen synthase and pyruvate dehydrogenase (the latter only in adipose tissue).

the mitochondrial ratio of [acetyl CoA]/[CoA] in muscles consequent upon oxidation of fatty acids and ketone bodies which inhibits pyruvate dehydrogenase directly, and phosphofructo-1-kinase and hexokinase indirectly via elevated concentrations of citrate and glucose 6-phosphate respectively (Fig. 3.3). For a recent review of the glucose/fatty acid cycle see Randle *et al.* (1988).

Based on the glucose/fatty acid cycle hypothesis, it has been suggested that insulin could exert its effect of stimulation of glucose utilization in muscle indirectly via its effects on lipolysis in adipose tissue (see for instance Newsholme, 1976; Espinal *et al.*, 1983). According to this proposal an important physiological role of insulin (with respect to glucose utilization) is its inhibition of lipolysis in adipose tissue. This will result in lowering of the plasma fatty acid concentration and hence

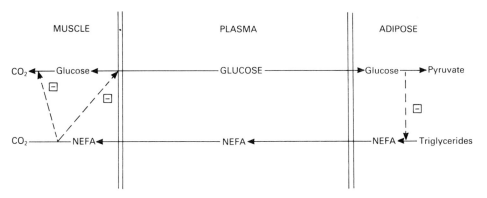

Fig. 3.2 — The glucose/fatty acid cycle.

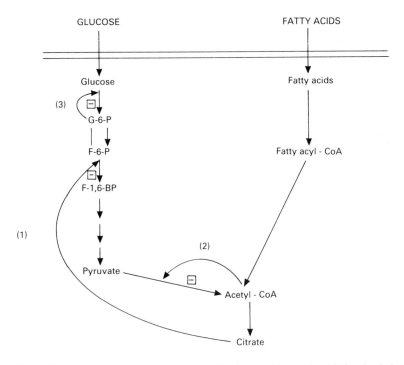

Fig. 3.3 — Mechanisms of control of glucose utilization by fatty acid oxidation in skeletal muscle. (1) Citrate inhibits phosphofructo-1-kinase. (2) Pyruvate dehydrogenase is inhibited by an increased ratio of [acetyl CoA]/[CoA]. (3) Hexokinase is inhibited by an increased concentration of glucose 6-phosphate (G 6-P). F-6-P, fructose 6-phosphate; F-1,6-BP, fructose 1,6-biophosphate.

the removal of the inhibition that the fatty acids exert on glucose utilization in muscle via their inhibition of pyruvate dehydrogenase. For this mechanism to operate *in vivo* it is necessary that adipose tissue be more sensitive† to insulin than muscle. This has been shown to be the case by several authors and a typical response is presented in Fig. 3.4. The amount of insulin needed to produce a half-maximal stimulation of

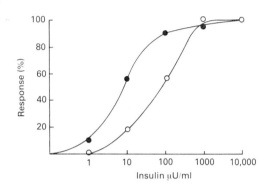

Fig. 3.4 — Comparison of the sensitivities of muscle and adipose tissue to insulin. (○) Skeletal muscle; (●) adipose tissue. Data taken from the author's D. Phil. thesis (University of Oxford).

glucose uptake in adipose tissue (10 μU/ml) is in the physiological range of insulin concentrations and is about an order of magnitude greater than that of muscle. It is important to stress that this indirect mechanism of insulin action only occurs in normal sedentary conditions when carbohydrate stores (i.e. glycogen) are full. Changes in the metabolic profile, for instance by sudden exercise, will cause dramatic changes in the sensitivity of a tissue to insulin.

The argument just presented may also offer an explanation for the observation that insulin does not cause a direct stimulation of pyruvate dehydrogenase in skeletal muscle but does so in adipose tissue. *In vitro,* and within ten minutes or so, insulin causes a 1.5- to 2-fold increase in the activity of pyruvate dehydrogenase in rat adipocytes. This rapid effect of insulin is thought to be directed to the conversion of glucose to fat after dietary intake of carbohydrate. No effects can be shown in muscle or heart, but in these tissues diabetes does cause a decrease in the activity of the enzyme which is reversible following treatment with insulin. These effects could also be explained by the changes in metabolite ratios caused by insulin following inhibition of oxidation of lipids. The effects of insulin on pyruvate dehydrogenase in adipose tissue could involve several factors and will be discussed in detail in section

† The clinical and pharmacological literature has had a long controversy concerning the use of the words 'sensitivity' and 'responsiveness' when describing the biological effects of a hormone. A definition suggested by many describes 'sensitivity' as referring to the concentration of a hormone required to produce half-maximal effects, and 'responsiveness' as referring to the maximal biological effect achievable by the hormone. I have attempted to maintain this usage of the terminology throughout the book.

4.2.3. However, a brief description may help the reader to understand the underlying mechanisms.

Pyruvate dehydrogenase is a mitochondrial enzyme complex that catalyses the irreversible oxidative decarboxylation of pyruvate to acetyl CoA according to the reaction:

$$CH_3COCOOH + NAD^+ + CoASH \rightarrow CH_3COSCoA + NADH + CO_2$$

The pyruvate dehydrogenase complex is regulated by product inhibition and through the concentration ratios of ATP/ADP, NAD^+/NADH and acetyl CoA/CoA. In addition, the complex is regulated by reversible phosphorylation; the phosphorylated enzyme is inactive and dephosphorylation will cause activation (Fig. 3.5). Insulin causes the conversion of phosphorylated (inactive) pyruvate dehydro-

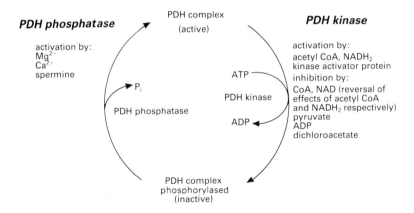

Fig. 3.5 — Regulation of the pyruvate dehydrogenase complex.

genase to dephosphorylated (active) enzyme. The mechanisms responsible for this are various and include the probable activation of pyruvate dehydrogenase phosphatase and the alteration in metabolite ratios caused by stimulation of alternate metabolic pathways (e.g. lipolysis and subsequent fatty acid oxidation by muscle). Further details are discussed below.

3.2.1.1.2   Glycogen metabolism
The control of glycogen metabolism in muscle is now well established and has been reviewed recently and extensively by Cohen *et al.* (1985). The two key enzymes which control the sysnthesis and breakdown of glycogen (glycogen synthase and glycogen phosphorylase, respectively) exist in interconvertible active and inactive forms. Phosphorylation gives rise to an increase in the activity of phosphorylase and a decrease in that of synthase. The active forms of the enzymes are designated by the

letter a and the less active ones by the letter b†., Phosphorylase b is dependent on AMP for its activity; it is stimulated by inorganic phosphate and inhibited by glucose 6-phosphate, ATP and ADP. Glycogen synthase b is dependent on glucose 6-phosphate and it is inhibited by ATP and inorganic phosphate.

The two enzymes are subject to a highly complex set of phosphorylation and dephosphorylation reactions catalysed by multiple kinases and phosphatases. Glycogen synthase may be phosphorylated by several kinases, including cyclic-nucleotide-dependent protein kinases, calcium-dependent protein kinases and at least four uncharacterized kinases. Phosphorylase is phosphorylated by phosphorylase kinase, which also phosphorylates glycogen synthase. Several non-specific phosphatases exist which dephosphorylate and phosphorylated enzymes (Fig. 3.6). The effect of

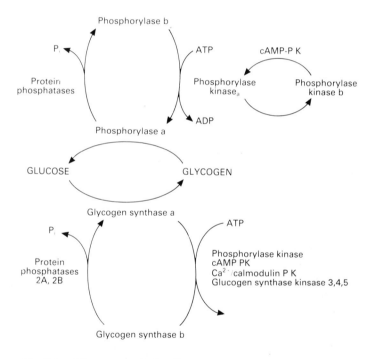

Fig. 3.6 — Glycogen metabolism in muscle. PK signifies protein kinase.

insulin on glycogen metabolism appears to involve activation of glycogen synthase by dephosphorylation of the enzyme, rather than inhibition of phosphorylase. The molecular mechanism for this effect involves inhibition of a glycogen synthase kinase and not activation of a phosphatase. These aspects will be discussed in detail in section 4.2.

---

† An accepted convention assigns the letters a and b to the active and inactive forms of proteins whose activity is regulated by reversible phosphorylation.

3.2.1.2 Liver
3.2.1.2.1 Glucose metabolism

Hepatic carbohydrate metabolism is highly complex because the liver has the capacity to utilize and make glucose, i.e. it is glycolytic and gluconeogenic simultaneously. This results in a complex set of regulatory mechanisms which for the most part are beyond the scope of this book. In most tissues glycolysis is related directly to glucose uptake. This is not the case in the liver. The transport of glucose in the liver is near equilibrium and once glucose is converted to glucose 6-phosphate several pathways may be taken. Moreover, the phosphorylation of glucose to glucose 6-phosphate is also different in the liver where it is catalysed by glucokinase, an enzyme possessing a K_m several orders of magnitude higher than hexokinase. The physiological implication of a high K_m (about 10 mM) is that the liver will only take up and phosphorylate glucose when its concentration is 10 mM or higher, which will only take place in circumstances such as ingestion of carbohydrates. The pathways of glycolysis and glycogen breakdown and synthesis are similar to those in other tissues. The main difference is the pathway of gluconeogenesis and its regulation. Gluconeogenesis, irrespective of the precursor (e.g. lactate, pyruvate, amino acids), appears to be controlled mainly and finely by hormones.

When the concentration of glucose in the blood increases, the secretion of insulin is increased and that of glucagon decreased. The opposite will occur when the plasma glucose concentration falls. Thus glucagon stimulates glucose formation whereas insulin inhibits it. These two hormones exert control of the gluconeogenic activity of the liver via the regulation of cAMP-dependent protein kinase (Fig. 3.7). Glucagon increases the concentration of cAMP in liver via stimulation of adenylate cyclase (see section 6.2). This results in activation of cAMP-dependent protein kinase and the subsequent phosphorylation of protein substrates for this kinase. In liver cAMP-dependent protein kinase phosphorylates pyruvate kinase and phosphofructo-2-kinase. The phosphorylation of pyruvate kinase results in a simple conversion of an active to an inactive form, thereby reducing the flux through glycolysis and increasing that through gluconeogenesis.

In terms of overall regulation of gluconeogenesis, the phosphorylation of phosphofructo-2-kinase is perhaps more important. A major development in recent years in the field of metabolic regulation was the discovery of fructose 2,6-biphosphate as an allosteric activator of phosphofructo-1-kinase and inhibitor of fructose 1,6-bisphosphatase. Fructose 2,6-bisphosphate is synthesized and degraded by a single bifunctional enzyme phosphofructo-2-kinase/fructose 2,6-biphosphatase (Fig. 3.8). The kinase activity of this enzyme is inhibited by citrate thus linking this mechanism to the regulation of glycolysis and the glucose/fatty acid cycle. In liver, the bifunctional enzyme is phosphorylated by cAMP-dependent protein kinase and dephosphorylated by protein phosphatase 2. Phosphorylation enhances the fructose 2,6-bisphosphatase activity of the bifunctional enzyme and dephosphorylation enhances its phosphofructo-2-kinase activity. This allows for coordinated regulation of glycolysis and gluconeogenesis by hormones such as glucagon. For reviews of this area the reader is referred to Hue & Rider (1987) and Pilkis et al. (1987).

Insulin antagonizes the effect of glucagon by lowering the concentration of cAMP in the liver once this has been elevated by glucagon. Insulin does not lower

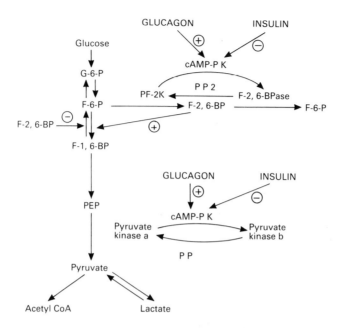

Fig. 3.7 — Hormonal regulation of gluconeogenesis. cAMP-PK signifies cAMP-dependent protein kinase; PP2 is protein phosphatase 2; PP is non-specific protein phosphatase; PF-2K is phosphofructo-2-kinase; F-2,6-BPase is fructose 2,6-bisphosphatase.

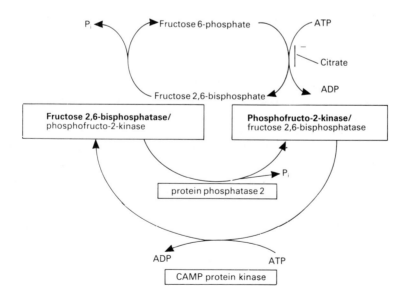

Fig. 3.8 — Regulation of phosphofructo-2-kinase/fructose 2,6-bisphosphatase.

basal cAMP levels. A fuller discussion of the relationship between insulin and glucagon, and of the insulin reversal of cAMP-mediated protein phosphorylation is presented in sections 4.2 and 6.2.

3.2.1.2.2   Glycogen metabolism

As in muscle, hepatic glycogen phosphorylase and synthase each exist in two interconvertible forms. The enzymes responsible for the phosphorylation and dephosphorylation processes are the same as in muscle, although fewer details are known about the liver enzymology than about that of muscle.

Insulin also promotes glycogen synthesis in liver and its effects are also due to the dephosphorylation of glycogen synthase. Insulin can activate glycogen synthase by counteracting the effects of glucagon and adrenaline on cAMP-mediated phosphory-lation and inactivation of the enzyme. The effect of insulin may be due to inactivation of a glycogen synthase kinase (as in muscle) or activation of a specific glycogen synthase phosphatase. The latter has been suggested on the basis of experiments that show *in vitro* effects of insulin that are independent of cAMP (see the review by Miller, 1985).

It is important to point out that hepatic glycogen metabolism may be regulated more by glucose concentrations than by hormones. It has been suggested that glucose itself may exert a regulatory influence on the activities of glycogen phosphor-ylase and synthase. As far back as 1877, Claude Bernard pointed out that 'cane sugar considerably increases the liver glycogen content', but he suggested the possibility that glucose produced this effect as a 'nutritive stimulator' rather than as a 'substance that is directly converted to glycogen' (Bernard, 1877). In recent times this proposal has once again been taken up in the form of the 'glucose paradox' hypothesis (see Katz & McGarry, 1984, for review). According to this hypothesis, only excessive glucose loads, which are rarely encountered by humans, are taken up directly by the liver. Instead, dietary carbohydrates are converted into liver glycogen indirectly via a sequence of reactions involving first of all the breakdown of glucose to three-carbon units (e.g. lactate). These three-carbon units are then taken up by the liver and converted to glycogen or fat. It is suggested that lactate is the best candidate for the three-carbon unit since it is known that glucose is converted to lactate in the gut and that muscle and red blood cells will also produce lactate from glucose. Thus, the metabolic flow is from lactate to glucose 6-phosphate and this is then diverted to glycogen instead of glucose. The mechanism for this would have to be either a direct inhibition by glucose of glucose 6-phosphatase or a stimulation (again by glucose) of glycogen synthase. Hepatic glycogen phosphorylase has a binding site for glucose. When glucose is bound, phosphorylase is dephosphorylated and hence inactivated. In addition, activated phosphorylase can inhibit glycogen synthase phosphatase. Therefore, glucose binding to phosphorylase can lead to the removal of this inhibition and hence to activation of glycogen synthase. This mechanism has not been conclusively proved but it does provide an explanation for a wealth of data.

3.2.2   Effects on fat metabolism

The major tissues for fat metabolism are white and brown adipose tissue and liver. The effects of insulin on fat metabolism in these tissues are qualitatively the same and I have therefore not divided this section according to tissue-specific effects.

Insulin increases the rate of fatty acid synthesis in white and brown adipose tissue, as well as in liver. In addition, the rate of triacylglycerol synthesis is also increased. In adipose tissue, insulin inhibits lipolysis. In contrast, lipogenesis is inhibited in liver by glucagon and in adipose tissue by adrenalin, i.e. by hormones that increase the concentration of cAMP. Thus, the key regulatory enzymes involved in the regulation of these pathways are finely controlled by hormones.

3.2.2.1 Fatty acid and triacylglycerol synthesis

The mechanisms responsible for insulin's effects appear to be the activation of pyruvate dehydrogenase (see above) and acetyl CoA carboxylase. Pyruvate dehydrogenase will provide acetyl CoA for conversion to fatty acids by the action of acetyl CoA carboxylase. In addition the sources for acetyl CoA will be endogenous lipolysis and fatty acids derived from the circulation. The regulation of pyruvate dehydrogenase was outlined above and will be discussed in section 4.2. Acetyl CoA is formed in mitochondria, but fatty acid synthesis occurs in the cytosol, and hence a mechanism is available for transport of acetyl CoA out of the mitochondria. Whilst long-chain acyl CoA may be transported via acetylcarnitine, the major mechanism for transport of acetyl CoA out of mitochondria is via the pyruvate/malate shuttle (Fig. 3.9). Once

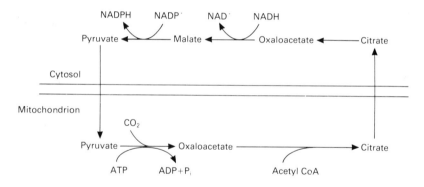

Fig. 3.9 — The pyruvate/malate shuttle.

acetyl CoA is in the cytosol it serves as a precursor for fatty acid synthesis. The first step in this long process (Fig. 3.10) (see Newsholme & Leech, 1983, for details) is the carboxylation of acetyl CoA catalysed by acetyl CoA carboxylase.

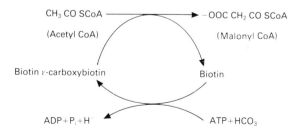

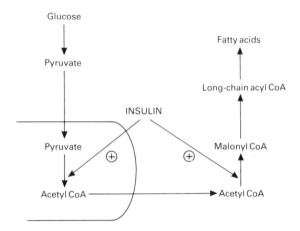

Fig. 3.10 — Sites of action of insulin on fatty acid synthesis.

Acetyl CoA carboxylase is the key regulatory step in the process of fatty acid synthesis. The enzyme can be isolated as a protomer of average molecular mass (M_r) 500 000, consisting of two identical subunits with an approximate M_r of 250 000. *In vitro*, acetyl CoA carboxylase can be converted to a polymer of M_r 5–20×10^6 which is active. The protomeric form of the enzyme has very low activity. Insulin increases the activity of acetyl CoA carboxylase by promoting its polymerization. In addition acetyl CoA carboxylase is also regulated by reversible phosphorylation with the phosphorylated form causing inactivation. Since one of the enzymes responsible for the phosphorylation of acetyl CoA carboxylase is cAMP-dependent protein kinase, those hormones that elevate the concentration of cAMP will cause inactivation of the enzyme. Interestingly, insulin actually causes the phosphorylation of acetyl CoA carboxylase; thus, controversy surrounds the possible role of reversible phosphorylation in controlling the polymerization process. Details of this will be discussed in section 4.2.3, but suffice it to say that insulin's stimulation of acetyl CoA carboxylase is one of the major mechanisms for the effects of the hormone on fat metabolism.

Insulin also appears to regulate the process of esterification of fatty acids to triacylglycerol, but the site of regulation is still unclear. It has been shown that insulin can increase the activity of glycerophosphate acyltransferase, the enzyme catalysing the acylation of a long-chain acyl CoA to the 1-position of glycerol 3-phosphate, which is the first reaction in the process of esterification of fatty acids (Fig. 3.11). This enzyme is also subject to regulation by reversible phosphorylation. In this case, cAMP-mediated phosphorylation causes inactivation and hence insulin's stimulation could be the result of its capacity to lower cAMP levels in liver.

3.2.2.2 *Triacylglycerol breakdown*
In the preceding discussion on the role and regulation of the glucose/fatty acid cycle, the importance of the insulin-stimulated inhibition of lipolysis in adipose tissue was emphasized. The key reaction in this process is catalysed by triacylglycerol lipase, also known as hormone-sensitive lipase. Indeed several hormones are known to

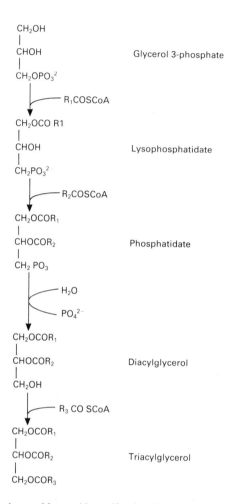

CH$_2$OH
|
CHOH   Glycerol 3-phosphate
|
CH$_2$OPO$_3^2$

— R$_1$COSCoA

CH$_2$OCO R1
|
CHOH   Lysophosphatidate
|
CH$_2$PO$_3^2$

— R$_2$COSCoA

CH$_2$OCOR$_1$
|
CHOCOR$_2$ Phosphatidate
|
CH$_2$ PO$_3$

— H$_2$O
— PO$_4^{2-}$

CH$_2$OCOR$_1$
|
CHOCOR$_2$ Diacylglycerol
|
CH$_2$OH

— R$_3$ CO SCoA

CH$_2$OCOR$_1$
|
CHOCOR$_2$ Triacylglycerol
|
CH$_2$OCOR$_3$

Fig. 3.11 — The pathway of fatty acid esterification. R represents a fatty acid chain.

affect the activity of this enzyme and they all appear to have their effects via changes in the concentration of cAMP. Hormone-sensitive lipase catalyses the hydrolysis of the ester links in triacylglycerol to yield fatty acids and glycerol. Hormone-sensitive lipase has long been known to be deregulated by reversible phosphorylation. Phosphorylation is catalysed by a cAMP-dependent protein kinase and results in the activation of the enzyme; dephosphorylation results in inhibition and is catalysed by a non-specific protein phosphatase. Thus hormones that increase cAMP via activation of adenylate cyclase (e.g. adrenalin, noradrenalin, glucagon, etc.) will stimulate lipolysis. Insulin inhibits lipolysis in part by lowering cAMP levels which is believed to be achieved by insulin stimulation of cAMP phosphodiesterase (Fig. 3.12).

Finally, an important enzyme of fat metabolism also regulated by insulin is lipoprotein lipase. Triacylglycerol is transported in the body in the form of chylomic-

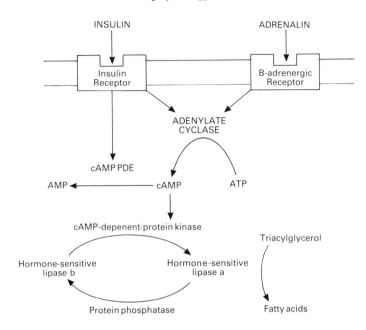

Fig. 3.12 — Hormonal regulation of lipolysis. cAMP-PDE, cAMP phosphodiesterase.

rons or other lipoproteins and cannot be taken up by any tissue in that form. It must be hydrolysed to fatty acids and glycerol, and this is the physiological role of lipoprotein lipase (Fig. 3.13). Perhaps due to its role, lipoprotein lipase is located in all tissues in the outer surface of the endothelial cells lining the capillaries and also in the plasma membrane of hepatocytes. The activity of lipoprotein lipase is also increased by insulin. The mechanism for this activation remained unknown until very recently when Saltiel and colleagues showed that lipoprotein lipase was anchored to the cell membrane via a glycosylphosphatidylinositol linkage and that insulin caused the cleavage of that linkage through stimulation of a phosphatidylinositol-specific phospholipase C (Chan *et al.* 1988). The significance of this finding relates directly to the current hypothesis of insulin action and will become apparent to the reader in subsequent chapters.

A different pathway that can be included in this sectin is cholesterol metabolism for its obvious associations with the metabolism of fats. The biosynthesis of cholesterol begins with the condensation of two acetyl CoA molecules to acetoacetyl CoA. This is converted to 3-hydroxy-3-methyl glutaryl CoA (HMG-CoA), which in turn is reduced to mevalonate by HMG-CoA reductase, in a reaction requiring NADPH. Then follow a series of reactions including phosphorylation, decarboxylation and condensations to yield cholesterol (the reader is referred to any textbook of metabolism for detailed examination of the steps leading to the formation of cholesterol). The key controlling enzyme in this process is HMG-CoA reductase, an enzyme also regulated by reversible phosphorylation. Phosphorylation of HMG-CoA reductase is catalysed by a specific kinase that is not cAMP-dependent;

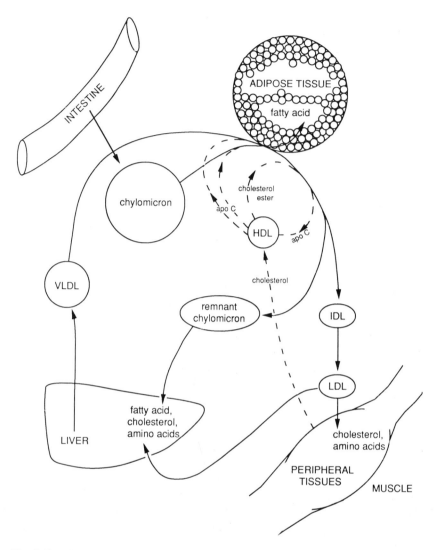

Fig. 3.13 — Schematic representation of lipoprotein metabolism. The diagram is reproduced from Newsholme & Leach (1983), by kind permission.

phosphorylation causes inactivation of the enzyme. The dephosphorylation is catalysed by a phosphatase similar to that which dephosphorylates glycogen phosphorylase. In addition to this interconversion, the kinase itself is also phosphorylated by another specific kinase, called HMG-CoA reductase kinase kinase, which is also cAMP-independent and which causes the activation of HMG-CoA reductase kinase. The phosphatase that dephosphorylates the reductase also dephosphorylates the kinase. Insulin increases the activity of HMG-CoA reductase although the mechanism by which this is achieved is unclear. Since phosphorylase phosphatase is inhibited by a protein (inhibitor-1) which itself can be phosphorylated and inhibited by cAMP-dependent protein kinase, it is possible that changes in cAMP may contribute to the effects of insulin. By analogy, glucagon causes the inactivation of HMG-CoA reductase.

3.2.3 Effects on protein metabolism
Insulin *in vitro* stimulates growth of cells in tissue culture. It is thought, however, that for the most part this effect is due to insulin binding to receptors for IGF-I and IGF-II. Nevertheless, in certain circumstances, insulin at physiological concentrations can increase cell division. Therefore, it has long been suggested, and indeed shown, that insulin can stimulate protein synthesis in a variety of tissues. In any given cell the concentration of a protein could be increased by several methods. The rate of synthesis of the mRNA coding for the particular protein or of the polypeptide chain by the ribosome–mRNA complex could be increased. Alternatively, the rate of degradation of mRNA or of the protein itself could be decreased.

Insulin stimulates the biosynthesis of many proteins including albumin, ATP–citrate lyase, acetyl CoA carboxylase, malate dehydrogenase, fatty acid synthase, glucose 6-phosphate dehydrogenase, pyruvate kinase, phosphoenolpyruvate carboxykinase, tyrosine aminotransferase, casein, amylase, and $\alpha_{2\mu}$-globulin. Insulin can also decrease the rate of protein degradation in skeletal muscle.

The metabolic effects of insulin on protein synthesis can be divided into rapid actions (those taking place over a space of minutes) and slower, long-term effects (taking place over hours). The rapid actions of insulin include stimulation of amino acid uptake, effects on translation factors and alterations in the phosphorylation state of proteins involved in protein metabolism. The slower effects are related to alterations in mRNA metabolism.

Insulin regulates the level of RNA in many tissues. These effects on transcription have been reported in liver, adipose tissue, pancreas and mammary gland. The effects of insulin could be due to increases in mRNA content, which has been shown for several of the enzymes listed above. In most tissues insulin can be shown to alter RNA levels, increase RNA polymerase and cause the phosphorylation of nuclear proteins. Direct effects of insulin on mRNA metabolism have also been reported, including mRNA efflux from nucleus and stimulation of nuclear nucleoside triphosphatase.

Finally, there is another possible target for insulin action related to protein metabolism. Ribosomal protein S6 is a component of the 40S subunit of eukaryotic chromosomes. Its role is unknown but it appears to be involved in the binding of mRNA. However, the relationship between phosphorylation and activity is unclear, although there are reports showing increased mRNA binding when there are increases in phosphorylation of S6. Insulin causes an increase in the phosphorylation of S6, but this has not been shown to be concomitant with an increase in mRNA binding. The role of this phosphorylation remains a mystery. Some further details concerning the reversible phosphorylation of S6 are presented in Chapter 4.

3.2.4 Summary
The effects of insulin on various metabolic pathways have been described and the molecular basis for these effects has been identified. The latter are summarized for

reference in Table 3.1. A common pattern emerges and that is that the effects of insulin on metabolic pathways are due to changes in the phosphorylation state of the key regulatory or controlling enzymes of each pathway. It becomes immediately apparent too that in the majority of cases the effect of insulin is to cause the dephosphorylation of enzymes. In addition insulin seems to cause the translocation of proteins within the cell (e.g. glucose carriers). The mechanisms whereby insulin causes these effects are the subject of Chapter 4. Before that it is necessary to consider the pathology of diabetes so as to appreciate the physiological role of the metabolic effects of insulin.

3.3 DIABETES MELLITUS

Diabetes is undoubtedly one of the major 'killer' diseases of Western countries. In the brief introduction to this chapter, I mentioned some of the compelling statistics surrounding the mortality of diabetes. In the United States, the National Commission on Diabetes estimates an annual increase in the incidence of diabetes of about 6%; adding this to the existing figure of 10 to 12 million diabetics, one can estimate that the size of the diabetic population in the United States will approach 20 million in the next few years. The annual cost of medical care of diabetic patients in the U.S. is currently estimated at $14 billion a year. The vast majority of this money is associated with treatments for the various complications of diabetes. As I mentioned above, diabetics are about 17 times more likely to develop renal failure, 25 times more likely to become blind, 20 times more likely to develop gangrene and twice as likely to develop heart attacks or suffer a stroke. Therefore, there can be little doubt of the severity of the disease and of the need for its treatment. However, in the absence of screening programmes, it is difficult to diagnose diabetics early enough to prevent development of complications. In fact most general practitioners tend to see a diabetic patient for the first time when he or she visits the doctor complaining of the symptoms of one of the long-term chronic complications of the disease.

Diabetes is not a single disease but a heterogeneous syndrome. Because of its heterogeneity it is difficult to give a general definition of the disease other than persistent and inappropriate hyperglycaemia. The U.S. National Diabetes Data Group has suggested a classification of diabetes into several types according to the origin of the disease. These are shown in Table 3.2 and correspond to the various definitions previously given in the literature such as chemical diabetes, latent diabetes, etc. The first type, spontaneous diabetes, represents 90% of all cases and it is divided into the two well-known types of diabetes: insulin-dependent or juvenile-onset diabetes, and non-insulin-dependent or maturity-onset diabetes. Within this group, between 85 and 95% of patients fall under the classification of non-insulin-dependent. The second group in Table 3.2 is secondary diabetes, described as the disease that arises from an insult to the pancreas, drug treatment, excess counter-regulatory hormones, or hyperglycaemia associated with a genetic syndrome. Impaired glucose tolerance refers to patients who have normal fasting plasma glucose levels but abnormally high glucose levels following glucose ingestion; this condition is occasionally referred to as chemical diabetes. Gestational diabetes refers to the abnormal glucose tolerance exhibited by some women during pregnancy.

Diagnosis of diabetes depends on the demonstration of hyperglycaemia or

Table 3.1 — Effects of insulin on metabolic pathways and target enzymes

Pathway	Enzyme	Effect of phosphorylation	Effect of insulin on enzyme activity	Effect of insulin on phosphorylation state	Proposed mechanism
Glucose transport	Glucose carriers	Unknown	Stimulation	Unknown	Translocation to cell membrane
Glycogen synthesis	Phosphorylase	Activation	Inhibition	Dephosphorylation	Decrease in cAMP?
Glycogen synthesis	Synthase	Inactivation	Stimulation	Dephosphorylation	Inhibition of specific kinase or activation of phosphatase
Gluconeogenesis	Pyruvate kinase	Inhibition	Stimulation	Dephosphorylation	Increase in protein synthesis decrease in cAMP?
	PF-2K	Inhibition	Stimulation	Dephosphorylation	Decrease in cAMP?
Glucose oxidation	PDH	Inhibition	Stimulation	Dephosphorylation	Activation of phosphatase
Fatty acid synthesis	ACC	Controversial	Stimulation	Phosphorylation	Polymerization
Esterification	GPAT	Inhibition	Stimulation	Dephosphorylation	?
Triglyceride transport	Lipoprotein lipase	None	Stimulation	None	Release from membrane
Lipolysis	HSL	Activation	Inhibition	Dephosphorylation	Decrease in cAMP?
Cholesterol biosynthesis	HMG-CoA reductase	Inhibition	Stimulation	Dephosphorylation	Decrease in cAMP?
Protein synthesis	S6	Activation	Stimulation	Phosphorylation	Activation of specific kinase

PF-2K, phosphofructo-2-kinase; PDH, pyruvate dehydrogenase; ACC, acetyl CoA carboxylase; GPAT, Glycerol-3-Phosphate Acyl Transferase; HSL, Hormone-sensitive lipase; HMG-CoA, 3-Hydroxy-3-methylglutaryl-CoA.

Table 3.2 — Classification of diabetes

1. Spontaneous diabetes mellitus
    (i) Type I or insulin-dependent diabetes (IDDM)
    (ii) Type II or non-insulin-dependent diabetes (NIDDM)

2. Secondary diabetes
    (i) Pancreatic disease
    (ii) Drug-induced
    (iii) Endocrine dysfunction (other than insulin)
    (iv) Genetic hyperglycaemia

3. Impaired glucose tolerance

4. Gestational diabetes

glucose intolerance. The diagnosis is usually made by measurement of the fasting blood glucose or by using the oral glucose tolerance test. An oral glucose tolerance test is performed by giving patients an oral glucose load of 75 g in 200 to 500 ml (or 1.75 g/kg weight for children) after an overnight fast of 10 to 16 hours, and measuring blood glucose over the following 2 hours. If the blood glucose concentration is equal to, or above, the levels indicated in Table 3.3, diabetes is diagnosed. Normally,

Table 3.3 — WHO criteria for diagnosis of diabetes

	Venous plasma glucose	Venous whole blood glucose	Capillary whole blood glucose
Fasting	>140 (7.8)	>120 (6.7)	>120 (6.7)
OGTT[a] (2 h)	>200 (11.1)	>180 (10.0)	>200 11.1)

Values are given in milligrams per decilitre; the figures in brackets are millimolar concentrations.
[a]OGTT, oral glucose tolerance test.

however, an oral glucose tolerance test is not necessary since most diabetics show fasting blood glucose levels over 7 mM. Once the diagnosis is made it is useful to classify the patients within the categories listed in Table 3.2. Since spontaneous diabetes comprises the vast majority of diabetics this will be the type discussed in this chapter. For a discussion of the clinical aspects of diabetes the reader is referred to Stanbury *et al.* (1983), Davidson (1986), Oakley *et al.* (1978) and many other clincally oriented textbooks.

3.3.1   Insulin-dependent diabetes mellitus (IDDM)

IDDM is the less common of the two types of spontaneous diabetes, representing less than 10% of all diabetics. As one of its descriptions implies, IDDM usually develops before 20 to 30 years of age and its onset is usually abrupt. This is in contrast to NIDDM where the disease manifests itself at 30 years of age or over, and where the onset of disease is very slow. A summary of the features of the two types of diabetes is presented in Table 3.4 for guidance and reference; the details are discussed below.

Table 3.4 — Features of Type I and Type II diabetes

	Insulin-dependent	Non-insulin dependent
Other definitions	Type I; juvenile-onset	Type II; maturity-onset
Proportion of diabetes	<10%	>90%
Age of onset	<30 years	>30 years
Appearance of onset	Acute	Slow
Response to insulin	Sensitive	Resistant
Tendency to ketosis	Very prone	Rare
Weight features	Loss of weight: wasting	Usually obese (>80%)
Treatment	Insulin; diet adjustment	Diet may be sufficient, oral hypoglycaemics, insulin not required
Pancreatic β-cells	Decreased	Normal or decreased
Plasma insulin	Decreased	Normal or elevated tendency to hyperinsulinaemia
Family history	Rare	Common
HLA association	Yes	No

3.3.1.1   Symptoms

Patients with IDDM usually present well-known symptoms, which include polyuria, thirst, tiredness, loss of weight associated with weakness, and drowsiness; the clinical picture also includes wasting, dehydration, glycosuria and ketosis. The onset of the disease may be very rapid, and symptoms such as loss or impairment of consciousness may occur before diabetes is diagnosed. The loss of weight is usually progressive but rapid weight loss of up to 10 kg (22 lb) in less than a month is not uncommon, and is always associated with polyuria. Following initial treatment with insulin, weight gain may be rapid and in addition the patients may suffer occasional hypoglycaemic episodes. Other symptoms include nocturnal enuresis in children and amenorrhoea. Occasional skin disorders are also observed such as pruritus vulvae and/or vaginitis, both of which are due to the combination of hyperglycaemia and glycosuria. The general symptoms of diabetes are equally applicable to both types of the disease, and thus the discussion of the details is kept within this section. The metabolic explanation for the symptoms is quite straightforward. Glycosuria is the result of the impairment in the glomerular absorptive capacity of the kidney, such that when plasma glucose is elevated it will appear in the urine. Polyuria and thirst (polydipsia) are the result of inhibition of water reabsorption in the kidney due to osmotic damage by glucose. Loss of body weight and wasting (both of which are only present in IDDM) is the result of breakdown of body fat and protein.

The most severe manifestation of type I diabetes is perhaps that of the diabetic coma, by which is meant a loss of consciousness due to uncontrolled diabetes. It arises due to severe diabetic ketosis. Patients with IDDM are far more prone to ketosis than those with NIDDM. Ketosis arises from the absence of insulin which leads to increased levels of plasma glucose and ketone bodies (due to lipolysis). Hyperglycaemia leads to polyuria, dehydration and loss of electrolytes. The increase in ketone bodies will lead to acidosis, vomiting and further dehydration and loss of electrolytes. All these manifestations will result in loss of consciousness. Diabetic coma is now rare, as it is prevented by accurate control with insulin. Prior to the discovery of insulin many diabetics died in coma. Thus the cause of IDDM is the absence of insulin.

3.3.1.2 Aetiology of IDDM
Destruction of the β-cells in the islets of Langerhans leads to insulin deficiency. The identification of the reasons for this destruction has been the focus of much research over the years. Present evidence indicates that genetic, environmental and autoimmune factors are involved in the aetiology of the disease. The familial incidence of IDDM is considerably lower than that of NIDDM. About 20% of IDDM patients have a relative who suffered the disease; the figure for NIDDM patients is as high as 90%. This suggests that environmental factors are involved in IDDM. However, a strong genetic component is suggested by the demonstrated increased frequency of certain histocompatability antigens (the HLA system) in patients with IDDM. The HLA antigens are glycoproteins present in the cell surface of all cells which are responsible for non-self recognition. The genes coding for the HLA antigens are located in chromosome 6, where they occupy four loci, designated A, B, C, and D. HLA antigens B8, Bw15, Dw3 and Dw4 are found with increased frequency in type I diabetics. Since the region of the HLA loci is close to that presumed to control immune responses, it seems likely that IDDM is the result of some disturbance of the immune system. There are several lines of evidence that suggest the involvement of an autoimmune process in the aetiology of IDDM. First, IDDM has long been associated with certain autoimmune disorders such as Addison's disease, Graves' disease, myasthenia gravis or pernicious anaemia. There have also been cases of mononuclear infiltrates in the islets of some type I patients. More importantly, 65 to 85% of patients have islet-cell antibodies at the time of diagnosis, although this figure decreases with time. These antibodies react with cytoplasmic determinants in the β-cell. The presence of the antibodies correlates with a progressive decline in insulin release prior to the development of diabetes. The current evidence therefore suggests that IDDM is a genetically determined disorder, mediated by autoimmune processes associated with some environmental insult. The autoimmune process results in the destruction of the β-cell and hence in insulin deficiency.

The evidence for the role of environmental factors in the aetiology of IDDM comes from several sources. Viruses are the most likely candidates to be the environmental factors. The frequency of diabetes associated with congenital rubella is as high as 20%. Several viruses can cause diabetes in animal models, but a genetic susceptibility appears necessary. A case has also been reported of a boy suffering a fulminant onset of IDDM following infection with Coxsackie virus B4. The virus, when isolated from the boy's pancreas, also induced diabetes in susceptible strains of mice.

Is it possible to unify these components of the aetiology of IDDM? A possible hypothesis is depicted in Fig. 3.14. A viral infection or other environmental insult may lead to partial damage to the β-cells. This may lead to the activation of B- and T-lymphocytes, a process which may be enhanced in susceptible individuals (e.g. those showing HLA association). An autoimmune process follows where the β-cells are recognized as non-self and destroyed, thus leading to insulin deficiency.

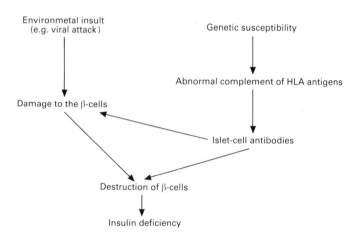

Fig. 3.14 — Aetiology of IDDM.

3.3.1.3 *Complications*

Diabetics who are well-controlled, that is their plasma glucose is kept within normal or near-normal levels, are nevertheless prone to a variety of life-threatening complications, which arise after many years of the disease and affect the arteries, capillaries, eyes, kidneys and nerves. As the percentage of diabetics dying of coma has decreased following the discovery of insulin from 60–70% to below 1%, the life-span of patients is much greater and this has been reflected in an increase in the appearance of the long-term chronic complications of diabetes. These conditions affect patients suffering from IDDM and NIDDM equally and therefore the aetiology of the diabetes has little to do with the aetiology of the complications. The importance of the diabetic complications cannot be overstated, as most diabetics die of premature heart attacks, kidney failure or stroke. Diabetic complications have been the subject of many reviews and books, so that what follows is a brief overview where the metabolic aspects of the complications will be discussed. The reader is referred to several clinical books such as Stanbury *et al.* (1983), Oakley *et al.* (1978), Dvornik & Porte (1987) for detailed discussion of these issues.

A common feature of diabetic complications is that they are related to the duration of diabetes and the degree of hyperglycaemia. Also treatment in the early stages of complications may help to prevent the latter stages, as there appears to be a point of no return in the development of the disease. Attempts to produce a common hypothesis for the origin of all the diabetic complications have yielded little success, but one theory has become popular in the last few years and has led to the development of a series of drugs for treatment (probably prophylactic) of diabetic complications.

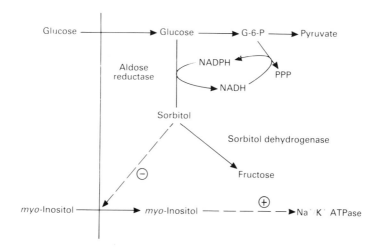

Fig. 3.15 — The polyol pathway of glucose metabolism.

The polyol pathway (Fig. 3.15) of glucose metabolism is not very active normally. The suggestion of the aldose reductase hypothesis is that in severe hyperglycaemia aldose reductase is activated and therefore sorbitol is accumulated. This leads to osmotic changes resulting in changes in membrane permeability and the onset of cellular pathology. The increase in tissue sorbitol levels results in a decrease in tissue *myo*-inositol (probably due to inhibition of *myo*-inositol uptake by sorbitol accumulation) and a decrease in the activity of Na^+/K^+ ATPase. Winegrad (see Winegrad, 1987) suggests that a decrease in the activity of this enzyme would result in abnormal nerve function, decreased glomerular filtration rate in kidney and derangements in the regulation of vascular tone. They suggest that the pool of *myo*-inositol that is inhibited by sorbitol accumulation regulates the activity of Na^+/K^+ ATPase. The proposed involvement of aldose reductase in the pathogenesis of diabetic complications has led to the identification of inhibitors of the enzyme. For a detailed discussion of these drugs and their possible therapeutic uses, advantages and disadvantages see the reviews by Kador *et al.* (1985) and Raskin & Rosenstock (1987).

Of all the diabetic complications, renal failure is the single major cause of death in patients with IDDM. Moreover, 25% of all end-stage renal failure can be accounted for by diabetic nephropathy. This condition is probably due to glomerular sclerosis. A common feature of diabetic complications is a thickening of the basement membrane. When this occurs in the glomerular capillaries there follows an impairment of the normal filtration properties of the capillaries, which will lead to proteinuria and a decrease in glomerular filtration rate. The progression of the disease can continue to the point where toxic end-products can accumulate in the blood and terminal renal failure ensues. Good glycaemic control may reverse the progression in the early stages of the disease, but later on other factors such as hypertension become important and may be key contributors to the mortality of this condition.

The incidence of retinopathy in diabetes is also very high, reaching close to 90% of diabetics after 20 years or more of the disease. Retinopathy is usually divided into non-proliferative and proliferative, although these represent different stages in the progression of the disease. Diabetic retinopathy is a disease of the microvasculature. Thickening of the basement membrane will result in larger small blood vessels, increased permeability and decreased capillary tonicity. Microaneurysms arise due to loss of pericytes and endothelial cell proliferation. These processes lead to development of new vessels, which extend from the retina into the vitreous humour, the appearance of secondary haemorrhages and eventual loss of vision. As with other diabetic complications, early diagnosis of diabetes may delay the onset of the retinopathy, but no specific therapy is currently available.

Diabetic neuropathy is probably as common as nephropathy or retinopathy, but because of the absence of direct objective clinical tests it is difficult to diagnose and to estimate its progression. The clinical picture of neuropathy is complex and includes cardiovascular (postural hypotension, resting tachycardia), gastrointestinal (diarrhoea, constipation, oesophageal atony) and urogenital factors (bladder atony, impotence, retrograde ejaculation, incontinence). In addition, peripheral nerve lesions, loss of sensation in the extremities, pains, paraesthesias are common. One of the classical syndromes occurring to diabetic patients, the 'diabetic foot', is an association of the peripheral neuropathy and microvascular problems with gangrene. The patient fails to notice damage to his or her feet, which can become gangrenous very quickly. The aetiology of diabetic neuropathy is unknown and no specific therapies exist.

Atherosclerosis in diabetics is as frequent as in non-diabetics, but diabetes accelerates the disease. It is difficult to establish the reasons for this but the abnormal fat and cholesterol metabolism and increased glycosylation of proteins may contribute to the process.

3.3.1.4   *Treatment*
The only treatment for IDDM is insulin, administered by injection usually twice per day. Clinical aspects of insulin administration may be found in the textbooks mentioned above.

In recent years, both islet and pancreas transplantation have become possible. This procedure is reasonably successful in animal models but few data exist in humans.

Another therapeutic approach under investigation is the antagonism of interleukin-1. Interleukin-1 is produced in monocytes and macrophages, and activates various cell types, such as B- and T-lymphocytes. Purified or recombinant interleukin-1 is cytotoxic to β-cells and can induce diabetes in animals. If interleukin-1 is involved in the aetiology of IDDM, antagonists to it may provide a useful therapy in the early stages of the disease.

3.3.2   Non-insulin-dependent diabetes mellitus (NIDDM)

NIDDM is the most common type of diabetes, affecting about 90% of patients. NIDDM appears in mid-life, usually around age 40 or over, and has a slow onset of symptoms. It is important to point out that the acute symptoms and the chronic complications of NIDDM are the same as in IDDM, with only a few exceptions. NIDDM patients rarely lose weight, but in fact do the opposite, and they are also rarely prone to ketosis. Thus the description of symptoms in section 3.3.1.1 and the discussion on complications in section 3.3.1.3 are applicable to NIDDM and will therefore not be repeated here.

3.3.2.1   Aetiology

Familial incidence of NIDDM can be present in as many as 90% of patients, yet the genetic component is less clear in this disease than in IDDM. A major reason for this is the total absence of an association with the HLA antigens. There is a strong component of environmental factors responsible for NIDDM such as age, diet, exercise and psychosocial stress.

The origins of the disease are uncharacterized but many factors appear to be present. Two groups of patients may be defined. In some cases insulin secretion is poor and the patients show severe fasting hyperglycaemia. In other cases insulin secretion is normal or even elevated and the patients show mild fasting hyperglycaemia. What is clear is that neither of these groups of patients respond to insulin: they are insulin-resistant. In addition the majority of NIDDM patients are obese. Both obesity and insulin resistance are heterogeneous diseases in which there is a diminished biological response to insulin, as shown in Fig. 3.16. The causes of insulin resistance may be varied and a few are discussed below.

A possible reason for the target cells not responding to insulin could be an abnormal insulin molecule. At least one such case has been reported in the literature. A defect or mutation in the insulin gene could be responsible for this modification.

A second possible cause involves the mechanism of insulin storage and secretion. A few cases have been reported where the patients show excess amounts of proinsulin and not insulin. It is worth noting, however, that these patients respond normally to exogenous insulin.

The presence of antibodies to both insulin and its receptor in the plasma of patients has been reported in the literature, and it is obvious that this would contribute to the development of the disease.

Finally, and most importantly, defects in the mechanism of action of insulin on its target cells are responsible for the pathogenesis of NIDDM. Since the mechanism of

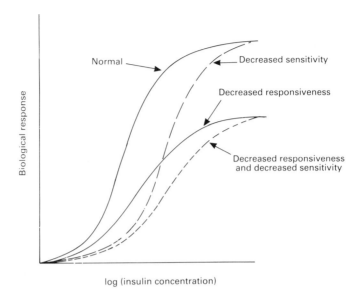

Fig. 3.16 — Insulin dose–response curves: sensitivity and resistance.

action of insulin is the main subject of this book, I shall not dwell at length on this point but present a brief overview with reference to NIDDM.

The mechanism of action of many hormones begins with the binding of the hormone to its receptor. This activates an effector enzyme which either directly or via the generation of a second messenger activates the target enzymes, thereby causing the physiological effects of the hormone. It is likely that all these steps are affected in NIDDM. Some patients exhibit a decrease in insulin binding to its receptor and/or a decrease in the number of functional insulin receptors. This kind of defect can be shown by a shift to the right in the insulin dose–response curve, with no alteration in the maximal response achievable. Thus the concentration of insulin now required to produce half-maximal effect is increased (Fig. 3.16). In some cases there is a defect at the post-receptor level. This may be due to a decrease in the effector enzyme activity, a decrease in the concentration of second messenger, a decrease in target enzyme activity or a variety of other possibilities. This defect is shown by a decrease in the maximal response achievable in response to insulin and hence in a shift downwards, and occasionally rightwards, in the dose–response curve. The latter case is usually more severe and other metabolic pathways (e.g. the glucose/fatty acid cycle) may be involved in the pathogenesis of NIDDM.

The identity of the primary lesion in NIDDM is a highly controversial topic. The primary candidates are peripheral insulin resistance, decreased insulin secretion and increased hepatic glucose output. It has been suggested that the increased glucose output could lead to hyperinsulinaemia and this in turn to insulin resistance. There are many reviews on this topic and I would recommend those by Olefsky *et al.* (1982), Flier (1983), Truglia *et al.* (1985), and Pershadsingh *et al.* (1986).

3.3.2.2 Treatment

Most NIDDM patients respond to therapy with diet alone or in combination with hypoglycaemic agents. The diet therapy involves restriction of dietary carbohydrates and fats. The currently available oral hypoglycaemic agents are the sulphonylureas. These compounds stimulate insulin secretion by the pancreas and have also been reported to increase glucose utilization by peripheral tissues, but the mechanism of action for this latter effect is not clear.

A therapeutic approach consists in the use of α-glucosidase inhibitors. These compounds inhibit carbohydrate absorption from the gastrointestinal tract by inhibiting α-glucosidase in the intestinal brush border. The compounds are capable of reducing post-prandial increases in blood sugar and reduce the fluctuations in blood sugar levels usually seen in diabetics.

REFERENCES

Bernard, C. (1877) *Leçons sur le diabète,* J. B. Baillière et fils, Paris.

Chan, B. L., Lisanti, M. P., Rodriguez-Boulan, E. & Saltiel, A. R. (1988) *Science* **241**, 1670–1672.

Cohen, P., Parker, P. J. & Woodgett, J. R. (1985) *Molecular basis of insulin action,* Czech, M. P. (Ed.), Plenum Press, New York, pp. 213–235.

Davidson, M. B. (1986) *Diabetes mellitus: diagnosis and treatment,* John Wiley & Sons, New York.

Dvornik, D. & Porte, D. (1987) *Aldose reductase inhibition: an approach to the prevention of diabetic complications,* McGraw-Hill, New York.

Espinal, J., Dohm, G. L. & Newsholme, E. A. (1983) *Biochem. J.* **212**, 453–458.

Flier, J. S. (1983) *Ann. Rev. Med.* **34**, 145–160.

Hue, L. & Rider, M. H., (1987) *Biochem. J.* **245**, 313–324.

Kador, P. F., Robinson, W. G. & Kinoshita, J. H. (1985) *Ann. Rev. Pharmacol. Toxicol.* **25**, 691–714.

Katz, J. & McGarry, J. D. (1984) *J. Clin. Invest.* **74**, 1901–1909.

Miller, T. B. (1985) In *Molecular basis of insulin action,* Czech, M. P. (Ed.), Plenum Press, New York, pp. 247–263.

Newsholme, E. A. (1976) *Clin. Endocrinol. Metab.* **5**, 543–578.

Newsholme, E. A. & Start, C. (1973) *Regulation in metabolism,* John Wiley & Sons, Chichester.

Newsholme, E. A. & Leech, A. R. (1983) *Biochemistry for the medical sciences,* John Wiley & Sons, Chichester.

Oakley, W. A., Pyke, D. A. & Taylor, K. W. (1978) *Diabetes and its management,* Blackwell Scientific Publications, Oxford.

Olefsky, J. M., Kolterman, O. G. & Scarlett, J. A. (1982) *Am. J. Physiol.* **243**, E15–E30.

Pershadsingh, H. A., Christensen, R. L. & McDonald, J. M. (1986) *Clin. Chem.* **32** (10 Suppl.), B19–B27.

Pilkis, S. J., Claus, T. H., Kountz, P. D. & El-Maghrabi, M. R. (1987) *The Enzymes* **18**, 1–46.

Randle, P. J., Garland, P. B., Hales, C. N. & Newsholme, E. A. (1963) *Lancet* **i**, 785–789.
Randle, P. J., Kerbey, A. L. & Espinal, J. (1988) *Diab. Metab. Rev.* **4**, 623–638.
Raskin, P. & Rosenstock, J. (1987) *Am. J. Med.* **83**, 298–306.
Stanbury, J. B., Wingerdan, J. B., Frederickson, D. S., Goldstein, J. L., Brown, M. S. (1983) *The metabolic basis of inherited disease,* Fifth Edition, McGraw, New York.
Truglia, J. A., Livingston, J. N. & Lockwood, D. H. (1985) *Am. J. Med.* **72**(2B), 13–22.
Winegrad, A. I. (1987) *Diabetes* **36**, 396–406.

4

Molecular mechanisms involved in insulin action

Many of the metabolic effects of insulin were shown in the previous chapter to be mediated via alterations in the phosphorylation state of the regulatory enzymes involved. In the majority of cases the effect of insulin is to cause the dephosphorylation of target enzymes. Thus, for instance, the key regulatory enzymes of glycogen synthesis (glycogen synthase), glucose oxidation (pyruvate dehydrogenase), lipolysis (hormone-sensitive lipase) are all dephosphorylated in response to insulin. It follows that dephosphorylation of regulatory enzymes is a central mechanism of insulin action.

Interestingly, insulin also causes the phosphorylation of various proteins including ribosomal S6 protein, ATP–citrate lyase and acetyl CoA carboxylase. In the majority of cases the phosphorylation can be described as silent; that is, it is unaccompanied by a change in the activity of the enzyme. It therefore appears that the mechanisms that lead to the phosphorylation of proteins in response to insulin may not be critical to the physiological actions of insulin.

Insulin has many other effects that do not appear to involve protein phosphorylation/dephosphorylation. Of these the stimulation of glucose transport is perhaps the best characterized. Insulin causes the translocation of glucose carriers to the plasma membrane, thereby increasing the amount of glucose going into the cell. The stimulation by insulin of protein movement, or traffic, within the cell is not confined to glucose transporters but includes the receptors for IGF-II and transferrin.

Finally, insulin causes changes in the expression of the genes for many proteins. At first glance many of these do not appear related to the metabolic effects of insulin. The mechanisms involved in insulin regulation of gene expression are poorly understood.

These topics are covered in the present chapter. I discuss only the effects of insulin on each of the enzymes involved and not their overall regulation; references to these topics will be given where required.

4.1   REGULATION OF PROTEIN PHOSPHORYLATION

The effects of insulin, or any other agonist, on the phosphorylation of proteins in intact cells can be studied by measuring changes in steady-state ^{32}P incorporation into protein. The methods employed by workers in this field are many, but typically, they include the prelabelling of cells with ^{32}P$_i$ in phosphate-free buffers, subcellular fractionation, and immunoprecipitation or gel electrophoresis to identify the proteins. These methods are generally applicable to the study of both phosphorylation and dephosphorylation, but the use of buffers that include inhibitors of kinases, phosphatases and proteases is widespread and recommended by many.

In considering the physiological importance of an effect of insulin on protein phosphorylation, it is worth employing the criteria suggested by Krebs & Beavo (1979) for assessing the role of reversible phosphorylation as a regulatory system. They suggested that an enzyme undergoes an physiologically relevant phosphorylation–dephosphorylation interconversion if:

(1) The enzyme can be shown to be phosphorylated *in vitro* by a specific kinase and dephosphorylated by a specific phosphatase.
(2) The functional properties of the enzyme undergo changes that correlate with the degree of phosphorylation.
(3) The enzyme can be phosphorylated and dephosphorylated *in vivo* or in an intact cell with accompanying changes in its functions.
(4) There is a correlation between the cellular levels of effectors of the kinase and phosphatase and the extent of phosphorylation of the enzyme.

When these criteria are applied, a list of proteins whose phosphorylation state is altered by insulin can be identified. This includes proteins that are phosphorylated and others that are dephosphorylated. These are discussed below.

4.1.1   Insulin-stimulated increases in protein phosphorylation
4.1.1.1   Acetyl CoA carboxylase
Acetyl CoA carboxylase catalyses the first regulatory reaction in the synthesis of fatty acids; namely, the conversion of acetyl CoA to malonyl CoA by the fixation of bicarbonate (see Chapter 3). Whilst this is not the only regulatory step in fatty acid synthesis, hormonal regulation of acetyl CoA carboxylase leads to regulation of that metabolic process.

Acetyl CoA carboxylase is found across several subcellular fractions in mammalian tissues, even though the cytoplasmic form of the enzyme is predominant. The active form of acetyl CoA carboxylase is a long filamentous polymer of M_r around 10^7. The protomer is composed of protomeric subunits which are dimers of identical subunits. The M_r of each subunit on SDS-PAGE (sodium dodecyl sulphate–polyacrylamide gel electrophoresis) is around 220 000–260 000. The variability in the subunit molecular weight appears to be due to the susceptibility of the enzyme to proteolysis, which can lead to loss of potential phosphorylation sites.

Acetyl CoA carboxylase is activated by citrate and inhibited by fatty acyl CoA esters. The activation by citrate is due to stimulation of polymerization, whereas fatty acyl CoA esters promote depolymerization. However, it is doubtful whether these processes have any physiological role. Thus, insulin activates the enzyme but there is no concomitant elevation of citrate levels or reduction of fatty acyl CoA esters. The same lack of correlation obtains with other hormones. Nevertheless, regulation of the enzyme's activity can indeed be achieved by the interconversion between polymerized and depolymerized forms. Thus, insulin is known to cause the polymerization of the enzyme.

Most current interest in the regulation of acetyl CoA carboxylase has focused on the role of reversible phosphorylation. The first demonstration of phosphorylation of the enzyme in intact cells was done using rat adipocytes (Brownsey et al., 1977). Studies on the effects of hormones have revealed that both insulin and adrenalin cause increases in the phosphorylation of acetyl CoA carboxylase in spite of their opposite effects on enzyme activity. Adrenalin causes a 50% decrease in activity of acetyl CoA carboxylase and a 40% increase in its phosphorylation. Insulin, on the other hand, causes a doubling of activity and yet increases phosphorylation of the enzyme by about 15% (Witters et al., 1979; Brownsey & Denton, 1982). However, two-dimensional thin-layer chromatography of peptides released by trypsin digestion of the enzyme reveals that the principal sites showing increased phosphorylation in response to insulin were different from those phosphorylated in response to adrenalin (Brownsey & Denton, 1982). These studies showing multisite phosphorylation of acetyl CoA carboxylase have been confirmed by other authors (Witters et al., 1983; Holland & Hardie, 1985).

The acetyl CoA carboxylase sites phosphorylated in intact cells in response to glucagon or adrenalin appear to be the same as those phosphorylated by cAMP-dependent protein kinase in cell extracts (Holland et al., 1985). It is therefore reasonable to suppose that the inhibition of fatty acid synthesis caused by adrenalin in adipose tissue and by glucagon in liver cells is mediated via activation of cAMP-dependent protein kinase, through the activation of adenylate cyclase by these hormones.

The effects of insulin remain controversial however. It is possible that an insulin-activated cAMP-independent protein kinase phosphorylates only one site that is different to that phosphorylated by cAMP-dependent protein kinase, and that phosphorylation of this former site correlates with activation of acetyl CoA carboxylase. The evidence for this has not been forthcoming. In fact, Haystead & Hardie (1986) showed that the effect of insulin on acetyl CoA carboxylase activity was lost on purification of the enzyme on avidin–Sepharose, whereas the effect on phosphorylation was not. These data suggested that phosphorylation and activation of the enzyme in response to insulin are separate and unrelated events. The authors also suggested that a low molecular weight effector mediates the activation of the enzyme by insulin.

Further recent controversy in this area has been produced by Witters and his colleagues. In a recent publication these workers have reversed their previous hypothesis and have presented evidence to show that insulin in fact causes the phosphorylation of acetyl CoA carboxylase (Witters et al., 1988). The authors also failed to observe a loss of enzyme activity during purification. Clearly, it would appear to an external observer that subtle methodological differences account for the radically different hypothesis now presented with respect to the effects of insulin on the phosphorylation of acetyl CoA carboxylase. It is at least clear that insulin does activate the enzyme, albeit through some uncharacterized mechanism.

4.1.1.2   Ribosomal protein S6

The ribosomal protein S6 is the major phosphoprotein of the eukaryotic ribosome 40S subunit. Its function is unclear, but appears to be associated with the binding of mRNA (Traugh, 1981). The phosphorylation of this protein occurs in at least five serine or threonine residues. Insulin stimulates the phosphorylation of S6 in various cell types (Smith *et al.*, 1979; Thomas *et al.*, 1980, 1982). Moreover, there is a strong correlation between the stimulation by insulin of protein synthesis and the level of phosphorylation of S6. This correlation, however, does not hold for other agents. Thus, agents that increase cAMP can cause the phosphorylation of S6 with no parallel changes in protein synthesis (Traugh, 1981). Early studies suggested that the sites phosphorylated via cAMP were different from those phosphorylated in response to insulin. However, more recent work suggests that the situation is far more complex. Whilst cAMP-dependent protein kinase is capable of phosphorylating two or three serine residues, insulin causes the phosphorylation of additional, mainly threonine, residues (Martin-Perez & Thomas, 1983; Martin-Perez *et al.*, 1984; Wettenhall & Morgan, 1984).

Much progress has been made in the identification of the protein kinase involved in the phosphorylation of S6 by insulin and other agents that also promote protein synthesis. Protein kinase C can phosphorylate some of the relevant residues in S6 (Parker *et al.*, 1985), but the most exciting development in this area is the report of the existence and purification of an S6-specific kinase (Erikson & Maller, 1985, 1986). This kinase has been purified to homogeneity from unfertilized *Xenopus* eggs. Erikson and co-workers have further characterized this kinase immunologically (Erikson *et al.*, 1987) and shown it to be present in various cell types. The kinase purified by these workers was termed by them S6 kinase II to distinguish it from another S6 kinase activity that can be co-purified and separated on Sephacryl chromatography. Two cDNAs have been isolated by hybridization to oligonucleotide probes designed to encode tryptic peptides isolated from S6 kinase II (Jones *et al.*, 1988). The cDNAs predict two proteins highly similar to each other containing two apparent kinase domains. The amino-terminal domain shows similarity to the ATP-binding and catalytic sites of protein kinase C, cAMP- and cGMP-dependent protein kinases. The other domain shows similarity to the ATP-binding site of the catalytic subunit of phosphorylase b kinase (Jones *et al.*, 1988).

Of great interest too is the observation that S6 kinase II can itself be regulated by reversible phosphorylation. Thus, *in vitro*, protein phosphatases 1 and 2A can deactivate S6 kinase II (Maller, 1987). On the other hand a number of serine/ threonine kinases, such as cAMP-dependent protein kinase and protein kinase C are unable to reactivate S6 kinase II. These observations suggested the existence of a kinase capable of activating S6 kinase II that was regulated by insulin. In a recent report, Sturgill and colleagues have shown that the insulin-stimulated microtubule-associated protein-2 (MAP-2) kinase phosphorylates and activates S6 kinase II

(Sturgill *et al.*, 1988). These experiments provide evidence for a step in the signalling of insulin involving the sequential activation by phosphorylation of at least two serine/threonine kinases.

4.1.1.3 ATP–citrate lyase
ATP–citrate lyase catalyses the formation of acetyl CoA from citrate in the cytosol, thereby leaving acetyl CoA in the right compartment for fatty acid synthesis. The enzyme exists as a tetramer of identical 123-kDa subunits and is phosphorylated at serine and threonine residues. Both insulin and hormones that elevate cAMP levels cause the phosphorylation of ATP-citrate lyase. Thus, phosphorylation of the enzyme is caused by agents that have opposite actions on fatty acid synthesis. In liver, both glucagon and insulin cause the phosphorylation of the same serine site. Furthermore this site is also phosphorylated by cAMP-dependent protein kinase (Pierce *et al.*, 1981, 1982).

In spite of the changes in phosphorylation state of the enzyme brought about by insulin, no concomitant changes in enzyme activity have been reported (Avruch *et al.*, 1985). Phosphorylation of ATP–citrate lyase has only been reported to cause a slight change in the affinity for ATP (Houston & Nimmo, 1985). Therefore, the present evidence suggests that phosphorylation of ATP–citrate lyase is a silent event; that is, it has no effects on the activity of the enzyme.

4.1.1.4 22-kDa protein
A 22-kDa cytoplasmic protein has been shown to be phosphorylated in response to insulin in rat adipocytes, 3T3-L1 cell, H4IIe cells and hepatocytes (Belsham *et al.*, 1982; Blackshear *et al.*, 1985; Vargas *et al.*, 1982). This protein is heat-stable and cannot be precipitated by 1 to 2% trichloroacetic acid. These peculiar characteristics are also shared by other proteins of similar size such as myosin light chains, inhibitor-1, and calmodulin. The electrophoretic pattern of this protein appears to change slightly with phosphorylation. Thus, phosphorylation of the 22-kDa protein is associated with a decrease in the phosphorylation of a smaller protein of similar characteristics. The two appear to be the same protein, migrating differently when phosphorylated. This protein can also be phosphorylated in response to EGF, PDGF, and serum (Blackshear *et al.*, 1983, 1985). The identity and function of the 22-kDa protein are unknown. Nevertheless, Denton and colleagues have suggested that it may initiate the dephosphorylation of other proteins in response to insulin by perhaps activating a protein phosphatase (Denton *et al.*, 1981).

4.1.1.5 46-kDa protein
A protein with $M_r = 46\,000$ is phosphorylated in response to insulin in freshly isolated hepatocytes (Avruch *et al.*, 1978; Vargas *et al.*, 1982; LeCam, 1982). It has not been found in adipocytes or other cells. However, it is not specific to insulin since, in addition to EGF, α-adrenergic agonists, glucagon and dibutyryl-cAMP can all cause the phosphorylation of this protein. Its identity and function are unknown.

4.1.2 Insulin-stimulated decreases in protein phosphorylation
Whilst the physiological role for the increases in protein phosphorylation discussed in the previous section is either unclear or controversial, the role for protein

dephosphorylation in the action of insulin is well-documented. In fact until evidence began to be accumulated that insulin caused increases in phosphorylation of certain proteins as well, it was widely held that all of insulin's actions were mediated through decreases in the phosphorylation of various enzymes.

The effects of insulin on the dephosphorylation of target proteins include cAMP-dependent and -independent mechanisms. It is well-known that insulin can reverse the cAMP-mediated phosphorylation of several proteins in liver and adipose tissue (Table 4.1). Thus, the inhibition by insulin of the activities of hormone-sensitive

Table 4.1 — Enzymes showing decreased phosphorylation in response to insulin

Enzyme	Tissues	Mechanism
Glycogen synthase	A,L,M	Unclear
HMG CoA reductase	L	Unclear
inhibitor 1	A,M	cAMP-mediated
Phenylalanine hydroxylase	L	cAMP-mediated
Phosphorylase kinase	A,L,M	cAMP-mediated
phosphorylase	A,L,M	cAMP-mediated
Pyruvate dehydrogenase	A,(L?)	Unclear
Hormone-sensitive lipase	A	cAMP-mediated

A, adipose tissue; L, liver; M, skeletal muscle.

lipase, pyruvate kinase, and phosphorylase kinase for example, can only occur if cAMP levels have already been elevated by β-agonists or other agents such as glucagon. The effect of insulin on these proteins does not appear to be due exclusively to changes in the concentration of cAMP but also includes a probable activation of phosphoprotein phosphatases. The molecular mechanisms involved in the effects of insulin on the levels of cAMP are covered in Chapter 6. Suffice to say here that the dephosphorylation of the enzymes listed in Table 4.1 occurs in part through a decrease in cAMP concentration, cAMP-dependent protein kinase activity, and activation of non-specific phosphatases.

The cAMP-independent effects are discussed below, and concern two enzymes of major importance in glucose homeostasis: glycogen synthase and pyruvate dehydrogenase. In neither case is the mechanism(s) involved in the activation by insulin of these two enzymes known, but both may involve the activation by insulin of specific phosphatases.

4.1.2.1 *Pyruvate dehydrogenase*
The pyruvate dehydrogenase (PDH) complex is a mitochondrial multienzyme complex catalysing the oxidative decarboxylation of pyruvate to acetyl CoA. The reaction is often described as the 'point of no return' for the glucose carbon, since the reaction is irreversible and the product provides substrate for the TCA (tricarboxylic acid) cycle or for fatty acid synthesis according to the tissue in which it occurs.

Reversible phosphorylation of the PDH complex appears to be the major regulatory mechanism of the activity of this complex, and hence of the rate of glucose oxidation in tissues. For reviews on the PDH complex see Randle (1986), Reed & Yeaman (1987), and Randle *et al.* (1988).

The PDH complex is composed of three enzymes (Table 4.2): E1 or pyruvate

Table 4.2 — Subunit composition of pyruvate dehydrogenase complex. The E1 component is the decarboxylase enzyme, E2 is the acyltransferase, and E3 is the dihydrolipoate dehydrogenase (see text for details)

Enzyme	Subunits		No. of subunits per complex
	Number	M_r ($\times 10^3$)	
E1α	2	41	60
E1β	2	36	60
E2	60	52	60
E3	2	55	12
Kinase α	1	50	
β	1	46	
γ	1	43	
Phosphatase I α	1	97	
β	1	50	
Phosphatase II α	1	60	
β	1	36	

dehydrogenase; E2, the acetyl transferase; and, E3, dihydrolipoyl dehydrogenase. The reaction catalysed by E1 is irreversible, and this confers irreversibility on the holocomplex reaction. The enzymes interact with one another through lipoate residues attached to a mobile arm in E2. This accepts a two-carbon product from pyruvate decarboxylation in E1 to form acetylhydrolipoate. Formation of acetyl CoA leads to the formation of dihydrolipoate from which H_2 is transferred to NAD by E3 (see Fig. 4.1). The PDH complex can be regulated through end-product inhibition via the reversal of the equilibrium reactions catalysed by E3 and E2.

The PDH complex is inactivated by phosphorylation catalysed by a specific kinase (PDH kinase), and activated by a specific phosphatase. PDH kinase is intrinsic to the complex (residing in E2) and co-purifies with it. On the other hand, PDH phosphatase can be readily separated from the complex during purification. As with the PDH complex, the kinase and phosphatase are also mitochondrial enzymes, and are hence regulated by mitochondrial effectors.

Phosphorylation occurs in serine residues at three different sites. Inactivation of PDH is largely due to phosphorylation of site 1. Phosphorylation of sites 2 and 3 appears to prevent the reactivation by PDH phosphatase. PDH kinase has been purified and is composed of three subunits: α (M_r=50 000), β (M_r=46 000), and γ

$$\underset{\text{O}}{\overset{\text{O}}{\text{RCCO}_2\text{H}}} + \text{CoASH} + \text{NAD}^+ \longrightarrow \underset{\text{O}}{\overset{\text{O}}{\text{RC}\sim\text{SCoA}}} + \text{CO}_2 + \text{NADH} + \text{H}^+$$

$(R=CH_3)$

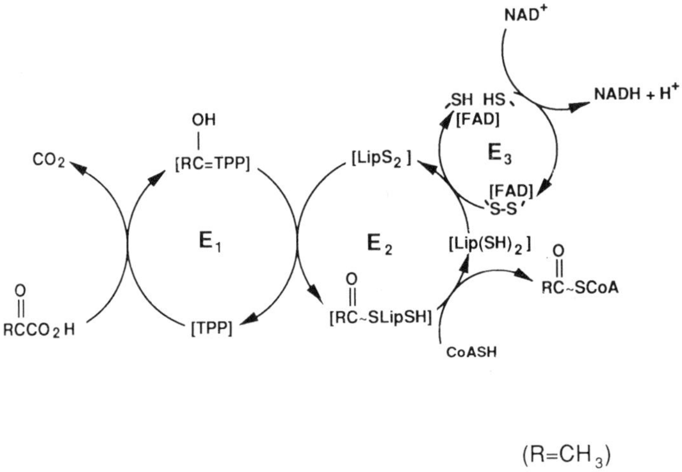

Fig. 4.1 — Reaction sequence of pyruvate dehydrogenase.

$(M_r=43\ 000)$. The α-subunit contains lipoate and may be a regulatory subunit, the β-subunit is the catalytic subunit, and the function of the γ-subunit is unknown (Stepp *et al.*, 1983). There appear to be two PDH phosphatases, which differ in their subunits but whose functional differences are unknown. Phosphatase I has two subunits: α $(M_r=97\ 000)$ and β $(M_r=50\ 000)$, whereas the α- and β-subunits of phosphatase II are 60 and 36 kDa respectively.

4.1.2.1.1 *Effects of insulin on the PDH complex*
In vitro, insulin rapidly increases the percentage of active PDH complex in rat adipocytes or fat pads. The maximum effect can be observed in 10 min and is generally about 1.5- to 2-fold (Denton *et al.*, 1971; Martin *et al.*, 1972). Very small short-term effects have also been reported to occur in hepatocytes, but the effects have been so small that they have proved difficult to reproduce. There are no rapid effects of insulin in skeletal or heart muscle PDH complex. It thus appears that in tissues where PDH has a anabolic role (synthesis of fatty acids) there is short-term regulation by insulin, whereas in those tissues where PDH has a catabolic role (muscle) there are no short-term effects of the hormone.

The effect of insulin persists during the preparation and incubation of intact mitochondria in the presence of an oxidizable substrate (Denton *et al.*, 1984). This property has been useful for many studies, and has revealed that the effects of insulin are not due to inhibition of PDH kinase but probably due to activation of PDH phosphatase. Recently, Denton and his colleagues have used toluene-permeabilized adipose tissue mitochondria to explore further these effects. Their studies appear to confirm that the major effect of insulin is the activation of PDH phosphatase (Thomas & Denton, 1986; Thomas et al., 1986).

The mechanism whereby insulin activates PDH phosphatase is, however, still controversial. PDH phosphatase may be regulated by Ca^{2+}, Mg^{2+}, and the NADH/ NAD$^+$ ratio. No increase in any of these regulators has been found in response to insulin. A very clear experiment by Denton and co-workers (Marshall et al., 1984) has shown that insulin did not cause an increase in mitochondrial Ca^{2+} concentration. Furthermore, the effects of insulin were restricted to PDH and did not include the other two Ca^{2+}-sensitive dehydrogenases, NAD–isocitrate dehydrogenase and oxoglutarate dehydrogenase. Interestingly, an increase in the activity of PDH phosphatase cannot be observed following exposure to insulin (Marshall et al., 1984; Thomas et al., 1986), suggesting that insulin may cause a change in the consentration of some effector of PDH phosphatase within intact mitochondria that dissociates during subsequent preparations. This effector could well be one of the putative second messengers for insulin that are discussed in Chapter 6. A further observation on the effects of insulin on PDH phosphatase is that they persist even in toluene-permeabilized mitochondria. In this system, insulin appears to cause an increase in the sensitivity of PDH to Mg^{2+}. These effects can be mimicked by spermine. In fact, spermine can be linked with the actions of insulin on the dephosphorylation of PDH and glycogen synthase, as well as having insulin-like effects on intact cells (Damuni et al., 1984; Tung et al., 1985). However, insulin does not cause changes in the concentration of spermine.

Long-term effects of insulin to reverse the effects of diabetes and starvation on inhibition of PDH activity have been reported to occur in perfused rat heart and in hepatocytes in tissue culture (Ohlen et al., 1978; Marchington et al., 1987). In the hepatocyte studies, the lower percentage of active PDH complex following starvation is maintained in culture for several hours and can be reversed by incubation with insulin, albeit at high insulin concentrations and long exposure (over 4 h). These effects of insulin may be associated with an inhibition of PDH kinase activity. It is unclear what physiological role these effects may have.

4.1.2.2 Glycogen synthase
Insulin stimulates glycogen synthesis in all its target tissues by the activation of glycogen synthase. Villar-Palasi & Larner (1960) showed that the enzyme existed in interconvertible forms and that the likely effect of insulin was to cause its dephosphorylation, since phosphorylation of glycogen synthase leads to its inactivation. Thus, a likely mechanism for this effect of insulin was the activation of a glycogen synthase phosphatase or the inhibition of a glycogen synthase kinase.

The work of Cohen and co-workers over the last few years has revealed that rabbit muscle glycogen synthase can be phosphorylated in as many as seven different serine sites by at least six different protein kinases (see Cohen, 1985, 1986, for reviews; see Table 4.3 for list). The seven phosphorylation sites are all contained in two cyanogen bromide peptide fragments, one at the N-terminus and the other at the C-terminal end of the protein (peptides CB-1 and CB-2 respectively, according to Cohen's nomenclature).

Both cAMP- and cGMP-dependent protein kinases phosphorylate the same sites

Table 4.3 — Glycogen synthase kinases

Kinase	Type of kinase	Sites phosphorylated
cAMP-dependent protein kinase		$1a > 2 > 1b$
	Cyclic-nucleotide-dependent	
cGMP-dependent protein kinase		$1a > 2 > 1b$
Phosphorylase kinase		2
Calmodulin-dependent multiprotein kinase	Ca^{2+}-dependent	$2 > 1b$
GSK-3		3a, 3b, 3c
GSK-4		2
GSK-5	Unspecified	5
Casein kinase-II		Six sites

(1a,2,1b). Phosphorylation by cAMP-dependent protein kinase is about 100 times faster than by its cGMP-dependent counterpart, and hence is likely to be of greater physiological significance. Phosphorylase kinase can phosphorylate glycogen synthase in addition to phosphorylating its usual substrate, phosphorylase. Phosphorylation of glycogen synthase by phosphorylase kinase is Ca^{2+}-dependent, as is that by calmodulin-dependent multiprotein kinase. Both phosphorylate the same residues (2 and 1b).

At least four uncharacterized kinases phosphorylate glycogen synthase at different sites. Glycogen synthase kinase 3 phosphorylates at sites 3a, 3b, and 3c. Kinase 4 phosphorylates at site 2, and kinase 5 phosphorylates at site 5. In addition, casein kinase-II can phosphorylate six sites. Glycogen synthase kinase 3 (GSK-3) has been purified from skeletal muscle; it has an M_r of 51 000 on SDS electrophoresis, but an M_r of 75 000 on gel filtration (Woodgett & Cohen, 1984). GSK-3 can phosphorylate itself and also the catalytic subunit of cAMP-dependent protein kinase, and casein. Glycogen synthase kinase 4 (GSK-4) appears to be highly specific for glycogen synthase, as no other protein seems to be phosphorylated by it. Glycogen synthase kinase 5 (GSK-5) is identical to casein kinase-II. The enzyme has been purified, and appears to be a heterodimer of $\alpha_2\beta_2$ composition, where the α-subunit has an M_r of 43 000 and the β-subunit an M_r of 26 000 (DePaoli-Roach et al., 1981). The enzyme has a broad substratre specificity and various unique properties, such as its ability to use GTP as well as ATP for substrate, inhibition by heparin and a 40-fold activation by polyamines. The relative ratios of GSK-3, GSK-4 and GSK-5 may be significant with respect to their physiological importance. GSK-3 accounts for about 90% of glycogen synthase kinase activity that is not cyclic nucleotide- or Ca^{2+}-dependent. GSK-4 accounts for about 7% and GSK-5 for less than 5% of the same activity.

Different phosphorylation sites have different effects on the activity of glycogen synthase; that is, phosphorylation at certain sites, but not others, causes inactivation of the enzyme. Phosphorylation of sites 3a, 3b, and 3c correlates with the loss of activity of the enzyme. A similar effect can be seen with phosphorylation at sites 2 and 1a. On the other hand, phosphorylation at sites 1b and 5 seems to have no effect on activity.

4.1.2.2.1   *Effect of insulin on glycogen synthase*

Insulin causes the activation of glycogen synthase and this is correlated with a decrease in the level of phosphorylation of the enzyme, even though the decrease is small (about 15%). The decrease in the amount of phosphate in the enzyme appears due to loss at sites 3a, 3b, and 3c; changes at other sites are not statistically significant. These data have been obtained from *in vivo* experiments (Parker *et al.*, 1983). In *in vitro* experiments the results are the same. Thus, Lawrence and colleagues have shown that only the cyanogen bromide peptide CB-2, which contains sites 3a, 3b, 3c, 5, 1a and 1b, loses phosphate in the presence of insulin (Lawrence *et al.*, 1983).

Therefore, insulin causes activation of glycogen synthase by promoting the dephosphorylation of sites 3a, 3b, and 3c. It follows that insulin will either activate protein phosphatases 1 or 2A, or inhibit glycogen synthase kinase 3. The current data available do not support either mechanism. The putative second messenger(s) for insulin may act by activating phosphatases, and this could be the way in which insulin activates glycogen synthase. Alternatively, Cohen and co-workers (see any of the reviews by Cohen cited) have suggested that the effect of insulin may be to inhibit GSK-3 by an, as yet, uncharacterized mechanism.

4.2   INSULIN REGULATION OF PROTEIN TRAFFIC

In the last few years it has become apparent that one of the ways in which insulin may cause some of its effects is by promoting the movement of target proteins within the cell. Insulin has been shown to cause this in at least three cases: the glucose transporter, IGF-II and transferrin.

4.2.1   Insulin stimulation of glucose transport

The stimulation of glucose metabolism by insulin in target tissues can be shown to be due to the stimulation of the transport of glucose into cells. This is probably the best-known effect of insulin and one directly linked to the hormone's ability to maintain normal plasma glucose levels. A large body of data exists on studies of glucose transport in adipose tissue, perhaps because of this tissue's exquisite sensitivity to insulin. Thus many of the current views on the effects of insulin on glucose transport have been derived from the original studies in adipose tissue by Kono and colleagues on the one hand, and Cushman, Simpson, and their colleagues on the other. Many reviews exist by these authors, and the reader is referred to them for a complete description of the work (Simpson & Cushman, 1985, 1986; Kono, 1985). What follows is an overview of the current hypothesis.

The stimulation by insulin of glucose transport occurs via an increase in the V_{max} of the process rather than a change in the K_m. Thus, there is an increase in the maximum rate of transport, rather than a change in the affinity for glucose of the transporter. The increase in maximum rate of transport could be due to an increase in the number of transporters. The stimulation of glucose transport by insulin occurs with a half-maximal stimulation at about 0.3 nM insulin; the maximal effect of insulin is at an upwards of 10–12-fold increase from basal levels.

Cushman and co-workers attempted to characterize the subcellular location of glucose transporters by using the binding of cytochalasin B to the transporter. Cytochalasin B is a fungal metabolite that is known to be a competitive inhibitor of glucose transport in human erythrocytes. It also interacts with other proteins, a problem that can be circumvented by using cytochalasin E to inhibit such interactions. Using this methodology, Cushman and co-workers showed that insulin caused an increase in the concentration of glucose transporters in the plasma membrane, without altering the K_d for the process. They were also able to show the presence of transporters in plasma membranes, and high- and low-density microsomes. In the presence of insulin, the concentration of transporters is increased in the plasma membrane fraction, unaltered in the high-density microsomes, and lowered in the low-density microsomes (Wardzala *et al.*, 1978; Cushman & Wardzala, 1980). Kono and colleagues reached the same conclusions using a different technique to assess the number of glucose transporters. In their assay the glucose transport activity is reconstituted into liposomes and the binding of labelled glucose is displaced with cytochalasin B (Suzuki & Kono, 1980; Kono *et al.*, 1981).

These and other data have led to the current hypothesis of the stimulation of glucose transport by insulin. The 'translocation hypothesis' suggests that following the binding of insulin to its receptors and the generation of a cellular signal, glucose transporters, which are normally located somewhere in the microsomal fraction, are translocated to the plasma membrane, where they fuse. The increased number of transporters leads to the increased rate of glucose transport (Fig. 4.2).

This hypothesis, initially proposed for adipose tissue, has been extended to other tissues (Wardzala & Jeanrenaud, 1981, 1983), and has been shown to be consistent with the changes in the sensitivity to insulin of glucose transport in animal models of insulin resistance (see the review by Simpson & Cushman, 1985, for details).

The glucose transporter from adipocytes has been purified and reveals a protein of about 45 kDa on SDS-PAGE. Recent data suggest that different glucose transporters exist in different tissues. Thus, using antibodies against the erythrocyte glucose transporter (M_r 55 000), Mueckler *et al.* (1985) cloned a transporter cDNA from human HepG2 cell line. This protein appeared identical to one encoded by a cDNA for the rat brain transporter (Birnbaum *et al.*, 1986). The data of James *et al.* (1988) suggest that the insulin-sensitive transporter may be different from these. Using monoclonal antibodies to the rat adipocyte transporter, they showed that only muscle and adipose tissue expressed this protein. Further support for this view may have been given recently by Thorens and colleagues, who have cloned a glucose transporter protein from rat liver that is expressed only in liver, kidney, intestine and in the β-cells of the pancreas, all of which are insulin-insensitive tissues (Thorens *et al.*, 1988).

Phorbol esters can stimulate glucose transport into cells and this appears to be due to stimulation of translocation of transporters (Kitagawa *et al.*, 1985). Since the erythrocyte glucose transporter can be phosphorylated *in vitro* and *in vivo* by protein kinase C, it has been suggested that phosphorylation of the transporter may be part

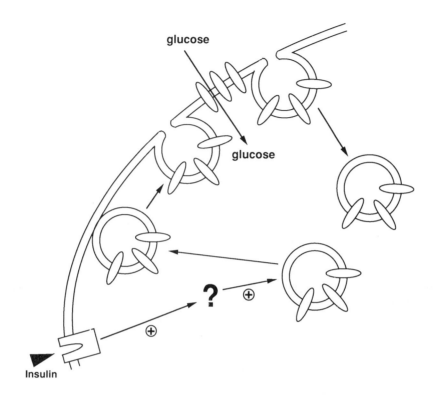

Fig. 4.2 — Translocation of glucose transporters.

of the signal involved in the translocation process (Witters *et al.*, 1985). However, insulin does not cause the phosphorylation of the glucose transporter in cells (Gibbs *et al.*, 1986).

4.2.2   Translocation of IGF-II receptors and other proteins
Insulin stimulates the appearance of IGF-II receptors at the plasma membrane of adipocytes (Oka *et al.*, 1984; Wardzala *et al.*, 1984). The hypothesis to account for this effect is essentially the same as suggested for glucose transporters; namely, the stimulation by insulin of the exocytosis of the receptors, as opposed to an inhibition of endocytosis.

It appears that insulin promotes the movement of non-phosphorylated IGF-II receptors, thereby decreasing the relative number of phosphorylated receptors at the plasma membrane (Corvera & Czech, 1985). The physiological relevance of these effects is unclear, but according to Corvera and Czech it suggests that phosphorylation of IGF-II receptors is a signal for their internalization (cf. insulin receptors in Chapter 5).

Insulin also causes the translocation of transferrin receptors to the plasma membrane. This appears to be a mechanism whereby insulin stimulates the uptake of iron into cells, a necessary requirement for growth (Corvera *et al.* 1986; Ward & Kaplan, 1986; Tanner & Lienhard, 1987).

It is interesting to speculate whether these translocations are specific or acciden-
tal. Is it possible that insulin causes the translocation of a specific intracellular vesicle
pool that happens to have in it glucose transporters, IGF-II receptors and transferrin
receptors, or are all these translocations tissue- or process-specific? The current data
have not answered this point.

4.3 REGULATION OF GENE EXPRESSION

The cellular effects of insulin can be classified according to the time of onset. Thus,
the vast majority of the metabolic effects of insulin occur within minutes following
binding of the hormone to its receptor. On the other hand, after hours or days insulin
has dramatic effects on cell growth associated with a large increase in protein
content. This increase has been associated with an increase in protein synthesis. For
certain enzymes the effect is to increase the amount of mRNA.

Several of the mRNAs regulated by insulin code for proteins with a clear
metabolic role. These include phosphoenolpyruvate carboxykinase, glucokinase,
fatty acid synthase, tyrosine aminotransferase, glyceraldehyde-3-phosphate dehydrogenase. Other mRNAs represent secretory proteins (albumin, growth hormone,
amlylase, $\alpha_{2\mu}$-globulin), proteins involved in reproduction (ovalbumin, casein), and
even structural proteins (δ-crystallin).

The mechanism by which insulin regulates the expression of any gene is unclear.
By analogy with other hormones affecting gene expression (e.g. oestrogen, glucocorticoids, prolactin), insulin could alter gene transcription, nuclear processing, cytoplasmic mRNA stability, or other factors.

The effects of insulin on the regulation of gene expression have only been studied
well in a few cases. Of these, the effects on phosphoenolpyruvate carboxykinase
(PEPCK) and glyceraldehyde-3-phosphate dehydreogenase (GAPDH) are amongst
the best described. The reader is referred to recent reviews by Granner and
colleagues (Granner et al., 1986) and Goodman and colleagues (Alexander &
Goodman, 1986). What follows is a summary of their observations without a
comprehensive review.

4.3.1 Effects of insulin on phosphoenolpyruvate carboxy-kinase (PEPCK) gene expression

PEPCK is a rate-limiting enzyme catalysing the conversion of oxaloacetate to
phosphoenolpyruvate, and as such plays a critical role in the regulation of gluconeogenesis (see Chapter 3). Glucagon, via cAMP, increases the rate of gluconeogenesis
and the synthesis of PEPCK. Insulin, on the other hand, decreases both (Beale et al.,
1981, 1985). The studies of Granner and his colleagues over the last few years have
led them to suggest that the effects of cAMP and insulin are to affect the production
of PEPCK mRNA, as opposed to any of the other possible mechanisms to increase
mRNA available. Glucocorticoids have the same effects as cAMP in this system.

The effects of insulin on the transcription of the PEPCK gene are rapid (achieved
in about 30–60 min), are achieved at physiological concentrations of the hormone,
and are clearly mediated through the binding of the hormone to its receptor. Insulin
appears to inhibit the basal rate of transcription of the PEPCK gene, suggesting
RNA polymerase II as a possible site of action. It is possible that the effects of
insulin, like those of cAMP, may involve the reversible phosphorylation of some

regulatory protein(s). The actual molecular mechanisms involved have not been elucidated.

4.3.2 Effects of insulin on glyceraldehyde phosphate dehydrogenase (GAPDH) mRNA

GAPDH is a glycolytic enzyme catalysing an equilibrium reaction. This makes it relatively unimportant from a regulatory point of view, except that regulation of its synthesis is of clear importance. Insulin increases the synthesis of this protein about four-fold, whilst the levels of its mRNA are increased about eight-fold. The effects are observed at near-physiological concentration of insulin, and are observed after exposure of cells to the hormone for 2 h. Few other details are available on this system.

REFERENCES

Alexander, M. & Goodman, H. M. (1986) In *Mechanisms of insulin action*, Belfrage, P., Donner, J. & Stralford, P. (Eds), Elsevier, Amsterdam, pp. 395–405.

Avruch, J., Witters, L. A., Alexander, M. C. & Bush, M. A. (1978) *J. Biol. Chem.* **253**, 4754–4761.

Avruch, J., Nemenoff, R. A., Pierce, M., Kwok, Y. C. & Blackshear, P. (1985) In *Molecular basis of insulin action*, Czech, M. P. (Ed.), Plenum Press, New York, pp. 263–297.

Beale, E., Katzen, C. & Granner, D. K. (1981) *Biochemistry* **20**, 4878–4883.

Beale, E., Andreone, T., Koch, S., Granner, M. & Granner, D. K. (1985) *Diabetes* **33**, 328–332.

Belsham, G. J., Brownsey, R. W. & Denton, R. M. (1982) *Biochem. J.* **204**, 345–352.

Birnbaum, M. J., Haspel, H. C . & Rosen, O. M. (1986) *Proc. Natl. Acad. Sci. USA* **83**, 5784–5788.

Blackshear, P., Nemenoff, R. A. & Avruch, J. (1983) *Biochem. J.* **214**, 11–19.

Blackshear, P., Witters, L. A., Girard, P. R., Kuo, J. F. & Quamo, S. N. (1985) *J. Biol. Chem.* **260**, 13 304–13 315.

Brownsey, R. W., Hughes, W. A., Denton, R. M. & Mayer, R. J. (1977) *Biochem. J.* **168**, 441–445.

Brownsey, R. W. & Denton, R. M. (1982) *Biochem. J.* **202**, 77–86.

Cohen, P. (1985) *Eur. J. Biochem.* **151**, 439–448.

Cohen, P. (1986) In *The enzymes,* Vol. 18, Krebs, E. G. & Boyer, P. D. (Eds), Academic Press, New York.

Corvera, S. & Czech, M. P. (1985) *Proc. Natl. Acad. Sci. USA* **82**, 7314–7318.

Corvera, S., Davis, R. J., Roach, P. J., DePaoli-Roach, A. & Czech, M. P. (1986) *Ann. N.Y. Acad. Sci.* **488**, 419–428.

Cushman, S. W. & Wardzala, L. J. (1980) *J. Biol. Chem.* **255**, 4758–4762.

Damuni, Z., Humphreys, J. S. & Reed, L. J. (1984) *Biochem. Biophys. Res. Comm.* **124**, 95–99.

Denton, R. M., Coore, H. G., Martin, B. R. & Randle, P. J. (1971) *Nature* **231**, 113–116.

Denton, R. M., Brownsey, R. W. & Belsham, G. J. (1981) *Diabetologia* **21**, 347–363.

Denton, R. M., McCormack, J. G. & Marshall, S. E. (1984) *Biochem. J.* **217**, 441–452.

DePaoli-Roach, A. A., Ahmad, Z. & Roach, P. J. (1981) *J. Biol. Chem.* **256**, 8955–8962.

Erikson, E. & Maller, J. L. (1985) *Proc. Natl. Acad. Sci. USA* **82**, 742–746.

Erikson, E. & Maller, J. L. (1986) *J. Biol. Chem.* **261**, 350–355.

Erikson, E., Stefanovic, D., Blenis, J., Erikson, R. L. & Maller, J. (1987) *Mol. Cell. Biol.* **7**, 3147–3155.

Gibbs, E. M., Allard, W. J. & Lienhard, G. E. (1986) *J. Biol. Chem.* **261**, 16 597–16 604.

Granner, D. K., Sasaki, K., Chu, D., Koch, S., Cripe, T. & Peterson, D. (1986) In *Mechanisms of insulin action,* Belfrage, P., Donner, J. & Stralfors, P. (Eds), Elsevier, Amsterdam, pp. 365–382.

Haystead, T. A. J. & Hardie, D. G. (1986) *Biochem. J.* **240**, 99–106.

Holland, R. & Hardie, D. G. (1985) *FEBS Lett.* **181**, 308–312.

Holland, R., Hardie, D. G., Glegg, R. A. & Zammit, V. A. (1985) *Biochem. J.* **226**, 139–149.

Houston, B. & Nimmo, H. G. (1985) *Biochim. Biophys. Acta* **844**, 233–239.

James, D. E., Brown, R., Navarro, J. & Pilch, P. F. (1988) *Nature* **333**, 183–185.

Jones, S. W., Erikson, E., Blenis, J., Maller, J. L. & Erikson, R. L. (1988) *Proc. Natl. Acad. Sci. USA* **85**, 3377–3381.

Kitagawa, K., Nishino, H. & Iwashima, A. (1985) *Biochem. Biophys. Res. Commun.* **128**, 1303–1309.

Kono, T. (1985) In *Molecular basis of insulin action*, Czech, M. P. (Ed.), Plenum Press, New York, pp. 423–433.

Kono, T., Suzuki, K., Dansey, L. E., Robinson, F. W. & Blevins, T. L. (1981) *J. Biol. Chem.* **256**, 6400–6407.

Krebs, E. G. & Beavo, J. A. (1979) *Ann. Rev. Biochem.* **48**, 923–959.

Lawrence, J. C., Hiken, J. F., DePaoli-Roach, A. A. & Roach, P. J. (1983) *J. Biol. Chem.* **258**, 10 710–10 719.

LeCam, A. (1982) *J. Biol. Chem.* **257**, 8376–8385.

Maller, J. L. (1987) *J. Cyclic Nucl. Prot. Phos. Res.* **11**, 543–555.

Marchington, D. R., Kerbey, A. L., Jones, A. E. & Randle, P. J. (1987) *Biochem. J.* **246**, 233–236.

Martin, B. R., Denton, R. M., Pask, H. & Randle, P. J. (1972) *Biochem. J.* **129**, 763–773.

Martin-Perez, J. & Thomas, G. (1983) *Proc. Natl. Acad. Sci. USA* **80**, 926–930.

Martin-Perez, J., Siegmann, M. & Thomas, G. (1984) *Cell* **36**, 287–294.

Marshall, S. E., McCormack, J. G. & Denton, R. M. (1984) *Biochem. J.* **218**, 249–260.

Mueckler, M., Caruso, C., Baldwin, S. A., Panico, M., Blench, I., Morris, H. R., Allard, W. J., Lienhard, G. E. & Lodish, h. F. (1985) *Science,* **229,** 941–945.

Ohlen, J., Siess, E. A., Loffler, G. & Wieland, O. H. (1978) *Diabetologia* **14**, 135–139.

Oka, Y., Mottola, C., Oppenheimer, C. L. & Czech, M. P. (1984) *Proc. Natl. Acad. Sci. USA* **81**, 4028–4032.

Parker, P. J., Caudwell, F. B. & Cohen, P. (1983) *Eur. J. Biochem.* **130**, 227–234.

Parker, P. J., Katan, M., Waterfield, M. D. & Leader, D. P. (1985) *Eur. J. Biochem.* **148**, 579–586.

Pierce, M. W., Palmer, J. L., Keutmann, H. T. & Avruch, J. (1981) *J. Biol. Chem.* **256**, 8867–8870.

Pierce, M. W., Palmer, J. L., Keutmann, H. T., Hall, T. A. and Avruch, J. (1982) *J. Biol. Chem.* **257**, 10 681–10 686.

Randle, P. J. (1986) *Biochem. Soc. Trans.* **14**, 799–806.

Randle, P. J., Kerbey, A. L. & Espinal, J. (1988) *Diab. Metab. Rev.* **4**, 623–638.

Reed, L. J. & Yeaman, S. J. (1987) In *The enzymes*, Vol. 18, Part B, Boyer, P. D. & Krebs, E. G. (Eds), Academic Press, New York, pp. 77–95.

Simpson, I. A. & Cushman, S. W. (1985) In *Molecular basis of insulin action*, Czech, M. P. (Ed.), Plenum Press, New York, pp. 399–422.

Simpson, I. A. & Cushman, S. W. (1986) *Ann. Rev. Biochem.* **55,** 1059–1089.

Smith, C. J., Wejksnora, P. J., Warner, J. R., Rubin, C. S. & Rosen, O. M. (1979) *Proc. Natl. Acad. Sci. USA* **76**, 2725–2729.

Stepp, L. R., Pettit, F. H., Yeaman, S. J. & Reed, L. J. (1983) *J. Biol. Chem.* **258**, 9454–9458.

Sturgill, T. W., Ray, L. B., Erikson, E. & Maller, J. L. (1988) *Nature* **334,** 715–718.

Suzuki, K. & Kono, T. (1980) *Proc. Natl. Acad. Sci. USA* **77**, 2542–2545.

Tanner, L. & Lienhard, G. L. (1987) *J. Biol. Chem.* **262**, 8975–8980.

Thomas, A. P. & Denton, R. M. (1986) *Biochem. J.*

Thomas, A. P., Diggle, T. A. & Denton, R. M. (1986) *Biochem. J.*

Thomas, G., Siegmann, M., Kubler, A. M., Gordon, J. & Jimenez de Asua, L. (1980) *Cell* **19**, 1015–1023.

Thomas, G., Martin-Perez, J., Siegmann, M. & Otto, A. (1982) *Cell* **30**, 235–242.

Thorens, B., Sarker, H. K., Kaback, H. R. & Lodish, H. F. (1988) *Cell* **55**, 281–290.

Traugh, J. A. (1981) In *Biochemical actions of hormones*, Litwack, G. (Ed.), Academic Press, New York, pp. 167–208.

Tung, H. Y. L., Pelech, S., Fischer, M. J., Pogson, C. I. & Cohen, P. (1985) *Eur. J. Biochem.* **149**, 305–313.

Vargas, A. M., Halestrap, A. P. & Denton, R. M. (1982) *Biochem. J.* **208**, 221–229.

Villar-Palasi, C. & Larner J. (1960) *Biochem. Biophys. Acta* **39**, 171–173.

Ward, D. M. & Kaplan, J. (1986) *Biochem. J.* **238**, 721–728.

Wardzala, L. J. & Jeanrenaud, B. (1981) *J. Biol. Chem.* **256**, 7090–7093.

Wardzala, L. J. & Jeanrenaud, B. (1983) *Biochem. Biophys. Acta* **730**, 49–56.

Wardzala, L. J., Cushman, S. W. & Salans, L. B. (1978) *J. Biol. Chem.* **253**, 8002–8005.

Wardzala, L. J., Simpson, I. A., Rechler, M. W. & Cushman, S. W. (1984) *J. Biol. Chem.* **259**, 8378–8383.

Wettenhall, R. E. H. & Morgan, F. J. (1984) *J. Biol. Chem.* **259**, 2084–2091.

Witters, L. A., Moriarty, D. & Martin, D. B. (1979) *J. Biol. Chem.* **254**, 6644–6649.

Witters, L. A., Tipper, J. P. & Bacon, G. W. (1983) *J. Biol. Chem.* **258**, 5643–5648.

Witters, L. A., Vater, C. A. & Lienhard, G. E. (1985) *Nature* **316**, 777–778.

Witters, L. A., Watts, T. D., Daniels, D. L. & Evans, J. L. (1988) *Proc. Natl. Acad. Sci. USA* **85**, 5473–5477.

Woodgett, J. R. & Cohen, P. (1984) *Biochim. Biophys. Acta* **788,** 339–347.

5

The insulin receptor

Many hormones and other extracellular stimuli exert their effects by binding to specific receptors on the plasma membrane of cells. The receptors recognize and bind the agonists with high affinity, and are therefore responsible for initiating the cascade of reactions leading to intracellular events. The hormone–receptor complex transmits this signal in various ways which are the subject of the next chapter, but which include interaction with a guanine-nucleotide-binding protein, activation of an effector enzyme, and generation of second messengers.

Insulin shares with other peptide hormones the prerequisite of a specific receptor on the membrane in order to transmit its effect. Ever since the original experiments of Cuatrecasas (1972a,b) there has been little doubt that insulin binds to a plasma-membrane receptor. Furthermore, the biological activities associated with the receptor have also been shown to be required for insulin action. These issues are discussed in this chapter.

5.1   RECEPTOR STRUCTURE

Over the last fifteen or so years many methods have been developed to examine and determine the structure of the insulin receptor. These methods have included the use of insulin bound to agarose (Cuatrecasas, 1972a,b), cross-linking radioactive insulin to plasma membranes and analysing the labelled proteins (Jacobs *et al.*, 1979), and the use of antibodies for precipitation of the receptor or in affinity chromatography techniques (see, for example, Jacobs & Cutrecasas, 1981). I will briefly review these methods since the first step in the elucidation of the structure of a protein has to be its purification.

5.1.1   Methods used in determining the structure of the insulin receptor

5.1.1.1   *Purification of the receptor*
The insulin receptor is a membrane-bound protein that comprises about 0.01% of total protein content in liver membranes. It is obvious, therefore that the first stage in purification should be a concentration of the starting source. The insulin receptor can

be solubilized with detergents such as Triton X-100 following a preparation of plasma membranes (Cuatrecasas, 1972a). A general scheme for receptor purification is shown in Fig. 5.1.

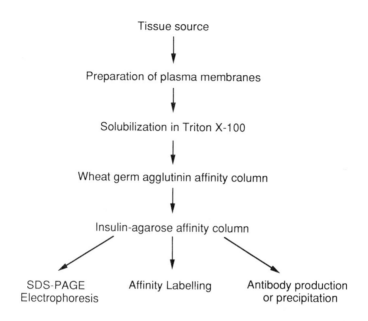

Tissue source

Preparation of plasma membranes

Solubilization in Triton X-100

Wheat germ agglutinin affinity column

Insulin-agarose affinity column

SDS-PAGE   Affinity Labelling   Antibody production
Electrophoresis   or precipitation

Fig. 5.1 — Flow diagram for purification of insulin receptor.

Following solubilization in Triton X-100, the insulin receptor can be further purified by the use of wheatgerm agglutinin (WGA) affinity chromatography. This technique uses the fact that both the α- and β-subunits of the insulin receptor are glycosylated and have N-acetylglucosamine residues in the carbohydrate structures. WGA has a high specificity for this sugar and hence the insulin receptor will bind to a Sepharose- or agarose-bound WGA. The receptor can be eluted off the column with 0.3-M N-acetylglucosamine, dialysed to remove the sugar and used for subsequent studies or for insulin–agarose affinity chromatography.

Insulin–agarose affinity chromatography was first described by Cuatrecasas (1972b). The principle is simple enough and is represented in Fig. 5.2. Insulin can be covalently attached to Sepharose beads by acylating native insulin with the N-hydroxysuccinimide ester of N-{3-[(3-aminopropyl)amino]propyl} succinamic acid--Sepharose. A column is packed with this material, and the solubilized membranes or the WGA eluant is passed through. Insulin receptors bind with high affinity to the beads, but other proteins pass through. Elution of the receptor off the column can be achieved with harsh conditions such as 4.5 M urea at pH 6.0, but these may lead to the denaturation of the receptor. For a full discussion of the methodology involved in purification and isolation of insulin receptors, the reader is referred to a recent book

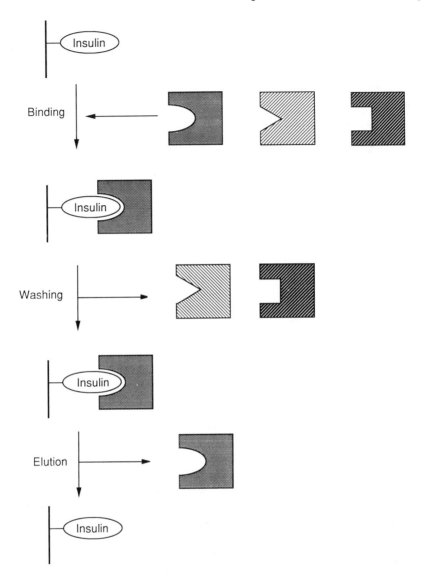

Fig. 5.2 — Affinity chromatography of insulin receptors.

on this topic (Kahn & Harrison, 1988). SDS-PAGE of insulin receptors purified by this method reveals three peptides of 135, 90 and 45 kDa, which correspond to the α- and β-subunits and a proteolytic fragment of the β-subunit (occasionally referred to as β1) respectively.

5.1.1.2 *Affinity labelling*
Insulin binding to its receptor is non-covalent and hence reversible. A major advance in the identification of the protein binding to insulin was the development of two

labelling techniques: photoaffinity labelling (see Yip, 1988, for review), and affinity cross-linking (Pilch & Czech, 1979).

Photoaffinity labelling is a very powerful technique used in many systems. The most frequently used photoreactive agents are the aryl azides. These agents are chemically stable in the dark, but if exposed to light they generate highly reactive free-radical nitrines that form covalent bonds with peptide chains. The efficiency is low, as a large proportion (up to 90%) does not cross-link covalently, but in spite of this the technique has proved very useful in the case of the insulin receptor. Here, insulin derivatives labelled with ^{125}I and containing an aryl azide group are synthesized so that they retain insulin-receptor-binding ability. They are incubated with membranes or purified receptors for an appropriate time and then photolysed, thereby achieving covalent binding.

Affinity cross-linking uses iodinated insulin, which is made to bind covalently to the receptor following an incubation period. The cross-linking is made possible by the addition of a bifunctional reagent capable of forming covalent bonds through two reactive groups. There are various techniques available for this methodology. On the whole, affinity cross-linking is more efficient in coupling, but photoaffinity labelling is more selective. In either case, the results obtained are similar. On SDS-PAGE a major band is revealed at 135 kDa, corresponding to the α-subunit of the insulin receptor. The β-subunit can occasionaly be detected as well.

5.1.2 Subunit composition

It is generally agreed that the insulin receptor is composed of two subunits: α, of 125–135 kDa; and β, of 90–95 kDa. The α-subunit was first identified by affinity chromatography and SDS-PAGE (Jacobs *et al.*, 1979) and subsequently by the cross-linking methods described above (Pilch & Czech, 1979; Jacobs *et al.*, 1979). Both the α- and β-subunits are glycosylated. This has been shown by the surface labelling of cells by the Hakomory procedure (sodium borohydride and galactose oxidase) (see Hedo, 1988).

The β-subunit, usually purified using the same techniques as for the α-subunit, is always stained less than the α-subunit on SDS-gels. It can also be labelled with carbohydrates on the extracellular domain. The β-subunit appears to be extraordinarily sensitive to proteolytic attack, as shown by the usual finding of fragments of 45–50 kDa found on SDS-gels. The β-subunit can also be labelled with γ-^{32}P-ATP under oxidizing conditions. The reason for this is the tyrosine kinase activity of the insulin receptor itself, which is located on the β-subunit (see below).

When insulin receptors are subjected to SDS-PAGE under non-reducing conditions, only one band is detected (at 300 kDa), which can be cross-linked with ^{125}I-insulin and if completely reduced yields the α- and β-subunits. These observations led both Jacobs and Cuatrecasas and Czech and colleagues to propose the currently accepted description of the structure of the receptor. This states that the insulin receptor is a heterodimer complex consisting of two α- and two β-subunits, with the β-subunits linked to the α-subunits through disulphide bridges, and the two α-subunits linked to each other in the same way (Fig. 5.3). Since both subunits are glycosylated and only the β-subunit has a hydrophobic domain, it is suggested that the β-subunit is the transmembrane subunit, whereas the α-subunit is extracellular.

Insulin-binding preparations of various molecular weights have been reported by

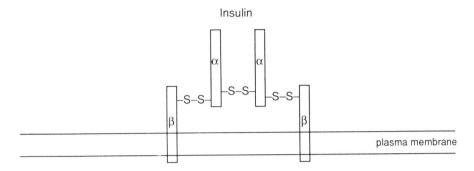

Fig. 5.3 — Schematic representation of the insulin receptor.

different authors and probably reflect the presence of different oligomers to the $\alpha_2\beta_2$ composition. Thus, oligomers of $\alpha\beta$ or α_2 have been described (Fujita-Yamaguchi, 1984).

5.1.2.1   *The insulin binding site*

The specific region within the α-subunit that insulin binds to had not been described until recently. In very recent experiments, DeMeyts and colleagues (DeMeyts *et al.*, 1988) suggest that insulin binds to a region containing the sequence Arg-Gly-Phe-Phe-Tyr. The argument presented is very provocative, as they propose that the binding domain of the insulin molecule and that of the region of the receptor to which it binds have exactly the same sequence! The significance of this is unclear at present but provides a novel concept of agonist–receptor interactions.

In another recent study Yip and colleagues have used a photoaffinity label on the insulin receptor to determine the region that insulin binds to (Yip *et al.*, 1988). The labelled α-subunit was cleaved by digestion with protease and revealed a band of 23 kDa. The authors provided evidence that the 23-kDa fragment contains residues 205–316 and that binding of insulin to its receptor occurs in the cysteine-rich region of the α-subunit. Thus, a synthetic peptide containing residues 243–251 bound insulin–agarose beads.

5.1.3   The insulin receptor precursor and its gene

The α- and β-subunits are derived from a common precursor of approximately 190–200 kDa (Massague & Czech, 1982). The precursor is synthesized in the endoplasmic reticulum and N-glycosylated on asparagine residues during transport to the Golgi apparatus. There it is cleaved to yield the α- and β-subunits and transfered to the plasma membrane.

A major advance in the knowledge of the structure of the insulin receptor and its relationship to other receptors came about in 1985, when two separate groups reported the sequence of the human insulin receptor cDNA. Both studies (Ullrich *et al.*, 1985; Ebina *et al.*, 1985) used the same approach and yielded the same data. The cDNA is shown in Fig. 5.4.

The insulin receptor precursor is a large molecule of 1340 amino acids in length, excluding the 27 amino acids of the signal peptide. The coding sequence is preceded by 50 nucleotides of 5′ untranslated sequence. A signal for translation termination and 1018 nucleotides of 3′ untranslated region follow the coding sequences.

The α-subunit is 719 residues long, is encoded for immediately following the signal peptide and is very hydrophilic. There are 15 potential asparagine-linked glycosylation sites, according to the consensus sequences for this process (-Asn-X-Ser/Thr-). The α-subunit contains 37 cysteine residues, 26 of which are located between residues 155 and 312, a highly hydrophilic region. These cytsteines are probably of importance in subunit interactions.

The β-subunit is 620 amino acids long, and contains four potential extracellular asparagine-linked glycosylation sites and four cysteine residues. It has a sequence of hydrophobic amino acids (915–940) that probably represents the transmembrane domain that anchors the receptor to the membrane. The intracellular region includes the region where the tyrosine kinase activity of the receptor resides.

The β-subunit follows the α-subunit in the cDNA sequence, and these are separated by a tetrapeptide sequence Arg-Lys-Arg-Arg, which is likely to be the recognition site for the precursor-processing enzyme. On the basis of this sequence the unglycosylated α-subunit would have an M_r of 82 500 and the β-subunit 69 700 (in reality 135 and 90 kDa respectively).

The insulin receptor gene is located on the short arm of chromosonme 19, appears to be 45 kilobases or greater in size, and seems to exist as a single copy in the human genome. A recent report has implicatd a polymorphism in this gene in the pathology of insulin resistance (McClain *et al.*, 1988). Few other studies of this type exist.

5.1.4   Relationship to other receptors

The insulin receptor shares homology with receptors for various other agonists. The homologies that exist can be of a structural or functional type as well as of primary sequence. Homologies exist between the insulin receptor and the receptors for IGF-1, EGF, low-density lipoprotein (LDL) and the cellular products of the oncogenes *v-ros* and *v-erb-B*. The greatest homology, of course, is with the receptor for IGF-1.

The insulin receptor α-subunit has a rich cysteine region that is similar to that found in other receptors such as EGF or LDL. It has been suggested (Ullrich *et al.*, 1985) that this region may form a functional domain such as the binding region for insulin. The insulin receptor has no primary sequence homology with the LDL receptor, and hence the homology with it is based on analogous domains. The insulin receptor has a wholly extracellular α-subunit that is cysteine-rich and is linked to the plasma membrane through its association with the β-subunit. The β-subunit has a membrane-spanning region and an intracellular domain. The LDL receptor, in contrast, has a similar structure in that there is a cysteine-rich region, a transmembrane domain, and an intracellular domain much shorter than that of insulin. In recent review articles, it has become popular to include a diagrammatic representation of these points and this is shown in Fig. 5.5.

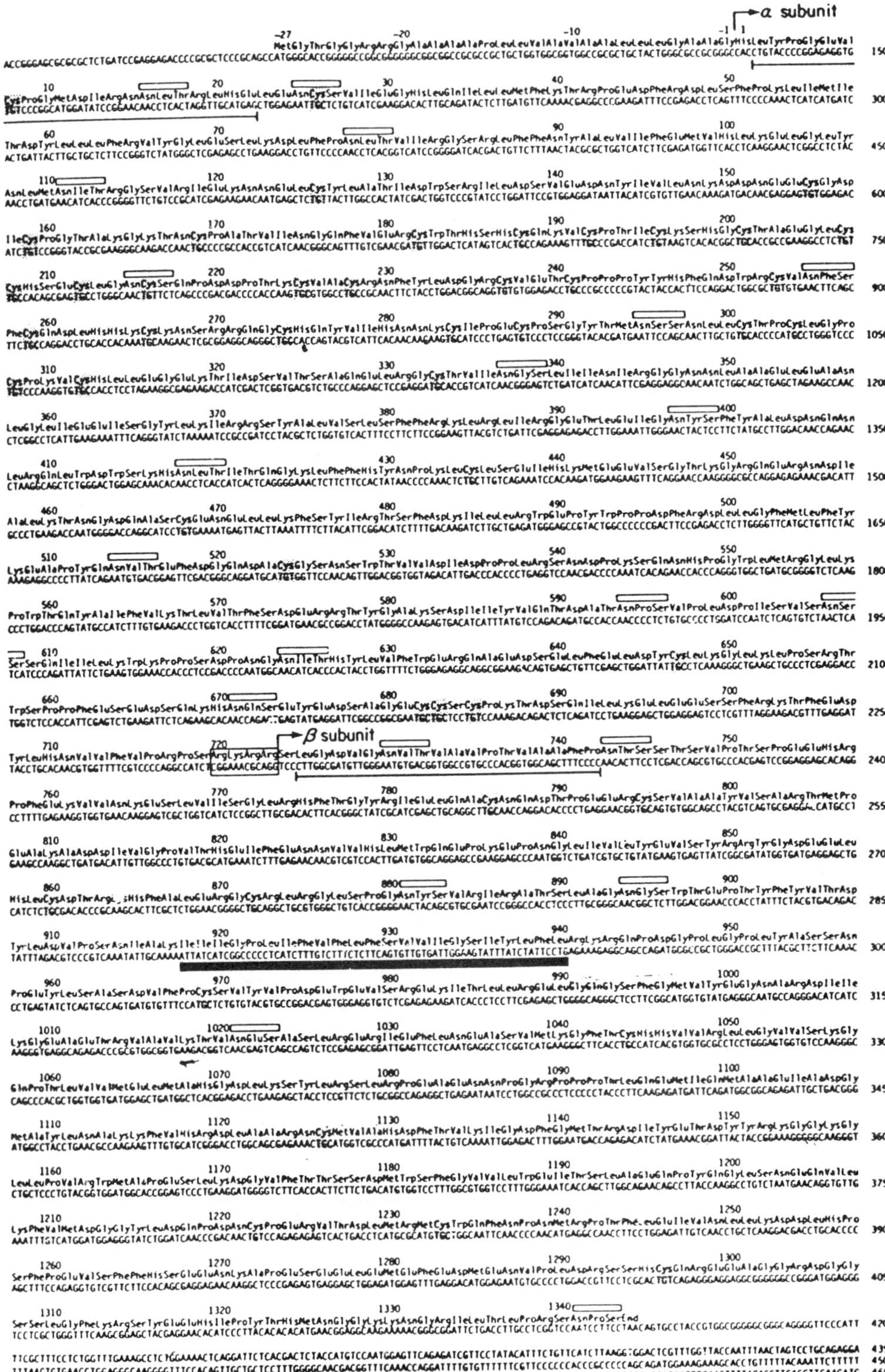

→ α subunit

```
                    -27                    -20                          -10              -1 1
                    MetGlyThrGlyGlyArgArgGlyAlaAlaAlaAlaProLeuLeuValAlaValAlaAlaLeuLeuLeuGlyAlaAlaGlyHisLeuTyrProGlyGluVal
ACCGGGAGCGCGCGCTCTGATCCGAGGAGACCCCGCGCTCCCGCAGCCATGGGCACCGGGGGCCGGCGGGGGCGGCGGCCGCGCCGCTGCTGGTGGCCGTGGCCGCGCTGCTACTGGGCGCCGCGGGCCACCTGTACCCCGGGGAGGTG   150

    10                  20                 30                 40                     50
    CysProGlyMetAspIleArgAsnAsnLeuThrArgLeuHisGluLeuGluAsnCysSerValIleGlyHisLeuGlnIleLeuLeuMetPheLysThrArgProGluAspPheArgAspLeuSerPheProLysLeuIleMetIle
    TGTCCCGGCATGGATATCCGGAACAACCTCACTAGGCTTGCATGAGCTGGAGAATTGCTCTGTCATCGAAGGACACTTGCAGATACTCTTGATGTTCAAAACGAGGCCCGAAGATTTCCGAGACCTCAGTTTCCCCAAACTCATCATGATC   300

    60                  70                 80                 90                     100
    ThrAspTyrLeuLeuLeuPheArgValTyrGlyLeuGluSerLeuLysAspLeuPheProAsnLeuThrValIleArgGlySerArgLeuPhePheAsnTyrAlaLeuValIleGluMetValHisLeuLysGluLeuGlyLeuTyr
    ACTGATTACTTGCTGCTCTTCCGGGTCTATGGGCTCGAGAGCCTGAAGGACCTGTTCCCCAACCTCACGGTCATCCGGGGATCACGACTGTTCTTTAACTACGCGCTGGTCATCGAGATGGTTCACCTCAAGGAACTCGGCCTCTAC   450

    110                 120                130                140                    150
    AsnLeuMetAsnIleThrArgGlySerValArgIleGluLysAsnAsnGluLeuCysTyrLeuAlaThrIleAspTrpSerArgIleLeuAspSerValAspAspAsnGluGlyGluGlyCysAsp
    AACCTGATGAACATCACCCGGGGTTCTGTCCGCATCGAGAAGAACAATGAGCTCTGTTACTTGGCCACTATCGACTGGTCCCGTATCCTTGATTCGGTGGATGATAATGAAGGTGACAACGAGGGTGGAGAC   600

    160                 170                180                190                    200
    IleCysProGlyThrLeuLysLysThrAsnCysProAlaThrValIleAsnGlyGlnPheValGluLeuArgCysLysGlnLysValCysProIleCysLysSerHisGlyCysThrAlaGluGlyLeuCys
    ATCTGTCCGGGTACCCTGAAGAAGACCAACTGCCCCGCCACCGTCATCAACGGGCAGTTTGTCGAACATGTTGGACTCATAGTCACTGCCCAGAAAGTTTGCCCGACCATCTGTAAGTCACACGGCTGCACCGCGGAAGGCCTCTGT   750
```

```
    210                 220                230                240                    250
    CysHisSerGluCysLeuGlyAsnCysSerGlnProAspAspProThrLysCysValAlaCysArgAsnPheTyrLeuAspGlyArgCysValGluCysProProProTyrTyrHisPheGlnAspTrpArgCysValAsnSer
    TGCCACAGCGAGTGCCTGGGCAACTGTTCTCAGCCCGACGACCCCACCAAGTGTGTGGCCTGCCGCAACTTCTACCTGGACGGCAGGTGTGTGGAGCACTGCCCGCCCCCGTACTACCACTTCCAGGACTGGCGCTGTGTGAACTTCAGC   900

    260                 270                280                290                    300
    PheGlnAspLeuHisHisLysCysLysAsnSerArgArgGlnGlyCysHisGlnTyrValIleHisAsnAsnLysCysIleProGluCysProSerGlyTyrThrMetAsnSerSerAsnLeuLeuCysThrProCysLeuGlyPro
    TTCCAGGACCTGCACCACAAATGCAAGAACTCGCGGAGGCAGGGCTGCCACCAGTACGTCATTCACAACAAGTGCATCCCTGAGTGTCCCTCGGGTTACACGATGAATTCCAGCAACTTGCTGTGCACCCCATGCCTGGGTCCC   1050

    310                 320                330                340                    350
    CysProLeuValHisLeuGluGlyGluLysThrIleAspTyrSerValThrSerAlaGlnGluLeuArgGlyCysThrValIleIleGlySerLeuLeuIleIleAsnIleArgGlyGlyAsnAsnLeuAlaAlaGluLeuGluAlaAsn
    TGTCCCCAAGGTGTGCACCTCGTAGAAGGCGAGAAGACCATCGACTATTCGGTGACGTCTGCCCAGGAGCTCCGAGGATGCACCGTCATCAACGGGAGTCTGATCATCAACATTCGAGGAGGCAACAATCTGGCAGCTGAGCTAGAAGCCAAC   1200

    360                 370                380                390                    400
    LeuGlyLeuIleGluGluIleSerGlyTyrLeuLysIleArgArgSerTyrAlaLeuValSerLeuSerPhePheArgLysLeuArgLeuIleArgGlyGluThrLeuGluIleGlyAsnTyrSerPheTyrAlaLeuAspAsnGlnAsn
    CTCGGCCTCATTGAAGAAATTTCAGGGTATCTAAAAATCCGCCGATCCTACGCTCTGGTGTCACTTTCCTTCTTCCGGAAGTTACGTCTGATTCGGGAAGAGACCCTGGAAATTGGGAACTACTCCTTCTATGCCTTGGACAACCAGAAC   1350

    410                 420                430                440                    450
    LeuArgGlnLeuTrpAspTrpSerLysHisAsnLeuThrIleThrGlnGlyLysLeuPheePheHisTyrAsnProLysLeuCysLeuSerGluIleHisHisMetGluGluValSerGlyThrLysGlyArgGlnGluArgAsnAspIle
    CTAAGGCAGCTCTGGGACTGGAGCAAACACAACCTCACTATCACTCAGGGGAAACTCTTCTTCCACTATAACCCCAAACTCTGTCTGAGTGAGATCCACCATATGGAAGAAGTTTCAGGAACCAAAGGGCGCCAGGAGAGAAACGACATT   1500

    460                 470                480                490                    500
    AlaLeuLysThrAsnGlyAspLysAlaSerCysGluAsnGluLeuLeuLysPheSerTyrIleArgThrSerPheAspLysIleLeuLeuArgTrpGluProTyrTrpProProAspPheArgAspLeuLeuGlyPheMetLeuPheTyr
    GCCCTGAAGACCAATGGGGACCAGGCATCCTGTGAAAATGAGTTACTTAAATTTCTTACATTCGGACATCTTTGACAAGATCTTTGAGATGGGGCCACTACTGGCCCCCCGACTTCCGAGACCTCTTGGGGTTCATGCTGTTCTAC   1650

    510                 520                530                540                    550
    LysGlnAlaProTyrGlnAsnValThrGluPheAspGlyGlnAspAlaCysGlySerAsnSerTrpThrValValAspIleAsproProLeuArgGlySerAsnAspProLysSerGlnAsnHisProGlyTrpLeuMetArgGlyLeuLys
    AAAGAGGCCCCTTATCAGAATGTGACGGAGTTCGACGGGCAGGATGCATGTGGTTCCAACAGTTGGACGGTGGTAGACATTGACCCCACCCTGAGGTCCAACGACCCCAAATCACAGAACCACCCAGGGTGGCTGATGCGGGGTCTCAAG   1800

    560                 570                580                590                    600
    ProTrpThrGlnTyrAlaIlePheValLysThrLeuValThrPheSerAspGluArgArgThrTyrGlyAlaLysSerAspIleIleTyrValGlnTyrAspAlaThrAsnProSerValProLeuGlnProIleSerValSerAsnSer
    CCCTGGACCCAGTATGCCATCTTTGTGAAGACCCTGGTCACCTTTTCGGATGAACGCCGGACCTATGGGGCCAAGAGTGACATCATTTATGTCCAGACAGATGCCACCAACCCCTCTGTGCCCCTGCAATCTATCAGTGTCTAACTCA   1950

    610                 620                630                640                    650
    SerGluSerGlnIleIleLeuLeuLysTrpLysProProArgAspAsnGlyAlaAsnIleThrHisTyrLeuValTrpGluGlnAlaGluAspArgGluLeuPheGluLeuAspTyrCysLeuLysLeuLeuLeuProSerArgThr
    TCATCCCAGATTATTCTGAAGTGAAACCACCTCCGACCCCAATGGCAACATCACCCACTACCTGGTTTTCTGGGAGCAGGCGGAGGACAGTGAGCTGTTCGAGCTGGATTATTGCCTCAAAGGGCTGAAGCTGCCCTCGAGGACT   2100

    660                 670                680                690                    700
    TrpSerProPheGluSerGluAspSerGlnLysHisAsnGlnSerGluTyrGluAspSerAlaGlyGluCysCysSerCysProLysThrAspSerGlnIleLeuLysGluLeuGluGluSerSerPheArgLysThrPheGluAspTyr
    TGGTCTCCACCATTCGAGTCTGAAGATTCTCAGAAGCACAACCAGTCTGAATATGAGGATTCCGCCGGGGAATGCTGCTCTTGCCCAAAGACAGACTCTCAGATTTTGAAGGAGCTGGAGGAGTCCTCGTTTAGGAAGACGTTTGAGGAT   2250
```

→ β subunit

```
    710                 720                730                740                    750
    TyrLeuHisAsnValValValProArgProProSerArgLysArgArgSerLeuGlyAspValGlyAsnValThrValAlaValProThrValAlaAlaGluThrGluLeuProSerArgProThrThrArgAsproProPheGluLysGluAspHisArg
    TACCTGCACAACGTGGTTTTCGTCCCCAGGCCATCCTCGAAAAGCAGCAGGTCTTGGGCGATGTTGGGAATGTGACAGTGGCCGTGCCTACCGTGGCAGCTGAGACCGAGCTGCCCAGCAGGCCCACCACAAGGGCTGGAGGAGCACAGG   2400

    760                 770                780                790                    800
    ProPheGluLysValValAsnLysGluSerLeuValIleSerGlyLeuArgHisPheThrGlyTyrArgIleGluLeuGlnAlaCysAsnGlnAspThrProGluGluArgCysSerValAlaAlaTyrValSerAlaArgThrMetPro
    CCTTTTGAGAAGGTGGTGAACAAGGAGTCGCTGGTCATCTCCGGCTTGCGACACTTCACAGGGTATCGCATCGAGCTGCAGGCTTGCAACCAGGACACCCCTGAGGAACGGTGCAGTGTGGCAGCCTACGTCAGTGCAAGGACTATGCCT   2550

    810                 820                830                840                    850
    GluLysAlaLysThrAlaAspAspIleValGlyProValThrHisGluIlePheGluAsnAsnValValHisLeuMetTrpGlnGluProLysGluProAsnGlyLeuIleValLeuTyrGluValSerTyrArgArgTyrGlyAspGluGluLeu
    GAAAAGGCCAAGGCTGATGACATTGTTGGGCCTGTGACGCATGAAATCTTTGAGAACAACGTCGTCCACTTGATGTGGCAGGAGCCGAAGGAGCCCAATGGTCTCATCGTGTTATATGAAGTGAGTTATCGGCGATATGGTGATGAGGAGCTG   2700

    860                 870                880                890                    900
    HisLeuCysAspAspThrArg...HisPheAlaLeuGluArgGlyCysArgLeuArgGlyLeuSerProGlyAsnTyrSerValArgIleArgAlaThrSerLeuAlaGlyAsnGlySerTrpThrGluProThrTyrPheTyrValThrAsp
    CATCTCTGCGACGACACCCGCAAGCACTTCGCTCTGGAACGGGGCTGCAGGCTGCGTGGCCTGTCACCCGGGAACTACAGCGTGCGAATCCGGGCCACCTCCCTTGCGGGCAACGGCTCTTGGACGGAACCCACCTATTTCTACGTGACAGAC   2850

    910                 920                930                940                    950
    TyrLeuAspValProSerAsnIleAlaLysIleIleIleGlyProLeuIlePhePheValPheLeuLeuSerValValIleLeuGlySerIleTyrLeuPheLeuArgLysArgGlnProAspGlyProLeuGlyProLeuTyrAlaSerSerAsn
    TATTTAGACGTCCCGTCAAATATTGCAAAAATTATCATCGGCCCCCTCATCTTTGTCTTCTCTCTCAGTGTTGTGATTGGAAGTATTTATCTATTCCTGAGGAAGAGGCAGCCAGATGGCCGCCGCTGGGACCGTTTACGCTTCTTCAAAC   3000

    960                 970                980                990                    1000
    ProGluTyrLeuSerAlaSerAspValPheProCysSerValTyrValProAspGluTrpGluValSerArgGluLysIleThrLeuLeuArgGluLeuGlySerPheMetValThrValGlyAlaArgAspIleIle
    CCTGAGTATCTCAGCGCCAGTGATGTGTTTCCATGCTCTGTACGTGCCCGACGAGTGGGAGGTGTCTCGAGAGAAGATCACCCTCCTTCGAGAGCTGGGCAGGTCCTTCGGCATGGTGTATGAAGGCCAATGCCAGGGACATCATC   3150

    1010                1020                1030                1040                   1050
    LysGlyGluAlaGluThrArgValAlaValLysThrValAsnGluSerAlaSerLeuArgGluArgIleGluPheLeuAsnGluAlaSerValMetLysGlyPheThrCysHisHisValValArgLeuLeuGlyValValSerLysGlyGln
    AAGGGTGAGGCAGAGACCCGTGTGGCAGTGAAGACAGTCAACGAGTCCGCCAGCCTGAGGGAGCGGATTGAGTTCCTCAATGAGGCCTCGGTCATGAAGGGCTTCACCTGCCATCACGTGGTGCGCCTCCTGGGAGTGGTGTCCAAGGGCCAG   3300

    1060                1070                1080                1090                   1100
    GlnProThrLeuValIleMetGluLeuMetAlaHisGlyAspLeuLysSerTyrLeuArgSerLeuArgProGluAlaGluAsnAsnProGlyArgProProProThrLeuGlnGluMetIleGlnMetAlaAlaGluIleAlaAspGly
    CAGCCCACGCTGGTCATCATGGAGCTCATGGCCCACGGAGACCTGAAGAGCTACCTCCGTTCTCTGCGGCCAGAGGCTGAGAAAATCCTGGCCGGCCTCCCCCTACCTTCAAGGAGATGATTCAGATGGCAGCAGAGATTGCAGACGGG   3450

    1110                1120                1130                1140                   1150
    MetAlaTyrLeuAsnAlaLysLysPheValHisArgAspLeuAlaAlaArgAsnCysMetValAlaHisAspPheThrValLysIleGlyAspPheGlyMetThrArgAspIleTyrGluThrAspTyrTyrArgLysGlyGlyLysGlyGly
    ATGGCCTACCTGAACGCCAAGAAGTTTGTGCATCGGGACCTGGCAGCGAGAAACTGCATGGTGGCCCATGATTTTACTGTCAAAATTGGAGACTTTGGAATGACCAGAGACATCTATGAAACAGACTACTACCGGAAAGGGGGCAAGGGT   3600

    1160                1170                1180                1190                   1200
    LeuLeuProValArgTrpMetAlaProGluSerLeuLysAspGlyValPheThrThrSerSerAspMetTrpSerPheGlyValValLeuTrpGluIleThrSerLeuAlaGluGlnProTyrGlnGlyLeuSerAsnGluGlnValLeu
    CTGCTCCCTGTACGGTGGATGGCACCGGAGTCCCTGAAGGATGGGGTCTTCACCACCTCTTCTGACATGTGGTCCTTTGGCGTGGTCCTTTGGGAAATCACCAGCTTGGCAGAACAGCCTTACCAAGGCCTGTCTAATGAACAGGTGTTG   3750

    1210                1220                1230                1240                   1250
    LysPheValMetAspGlyGlyTyrLeuAspGlnProAspAsnCysProGluArgValThrAspLeuMetArgMetCysTrpGlnPheAsnProAsnMetArgProThrPhe.GluIleLeuAsnLeuLeuLeuAspAspLeuHisPro
    AAATTTGTCATGGATGGAGGGTATCTGGATCAACCCGACAACTGTCCAGAGAGAGTCACTGACCTCATGCGCATGTGCTGGCAATTCAACCCCAACATGAGGCCCACTTTCGTTGGGAGATTCTCAACCTTGCTTCTTGATGATCTTCACCCC   3900

    1260                1270                1280                1290                   1300
    SerPheProGluValSerPhePheHisSerGluGluAsnLysAlaProGluSerGluGluLeuGluMetGluPheGluAspMetGluAsnValProLeuAspArgSerSerHisCysGlnArgGluGluAlaGlyGlyArgAspGlyGly
    AGCTTTCCAGAGGTTCGTTCTTCCACAGAGGAGAACAAAGCTCCCGAGAGTGAGGAGCTGGAGATGGAGTTTGAGGACATGGAGAATGTGCCTCTGGACAGGTCGTCGCACTGTCAGAGGGAGGAGGCGGGGGGCCGGGATGGGGGA   4050

    1310                1320                1330                1340
    SerSerLeuGlyPheLysArgSerTyrGluGluHisIleProTyrThrHisMetAsnGlyGlyLysLysAsnGlyArgIleLeuThrLeuProArgSerAsnProSer End
    TCCTCGCTTGGCTTCAAGAGGTCGTACGAAGAGCACATACCCTACACACACATGAACGGTGGGAAGAAAAATGGTCGAATCCTCACACTGCCTCGGTCCAACCCTTCTTAATGAGCTTCTACCGTGGCGGGGGAGCGGGGAGGGGTTCCCATT   4700
```

```
TTCGCTTTCCTCTGGTTTGAAAGCCTCTGGAAAACTCAGGATTCTCACGACTCTACCATGTCCAATGCAGTTCAGAGATCGTTCCTATACATTCTGTTCATCTTAAGCGGACTCGTTTGGTTACCAATTTAACTAGTCCTGCAGAGGA   4350
TTTAACTGTGAACCTGGACGGCAAGGGGTTTCACAGTTGCTGCTCCTTTGGGAGCCTCTGATGTCCTTTCAAACCAGGATTTTGTGTTTTTCTTGTTTCCCACCCGCCCCAGCAGGTCAGTTTTTTCCCACACCACCTTTTATGTCCTCAAGATG   4650
TTTTTTTTTTTTTGCTGGTTTTTTTTTTTTTAATAAAAGCAAAATTTCCTGTTTGTGGAACAAAATTCAAGTTTTACAAGTTGAGCTTCAAGATG   4800
GTTTTTTGGTTTTTTTCTCATTTACTGCTTGCTCTGGAAAACTGTTTTTTTCTTTACAAAATGAGTTCTCAATGAACAATAGCTGTTTCATATTTTCTGCTTCAGGTGCTCCTTCGTGTCCCGGCGTGTCAGGACTCATCCCCTCTCTCCTTCCTTCATTTGATCGTATT   4950
ACAGATTCTTCTTGTGTCAGAAGTCTAGCCTCAGTTTCTACCCTCCTTTCACATTGGTGGCCAAGGAGCATTCATTTGGAGTGATTATGATTTTCAAGACCAAACAAGCTAGGACATTAAAAAAAAAAAAAGAAAAAAG   5100
AAGCAAAAAACAAAATGGAAAAAGCAAAAAAGAAAAAAGAAACTGAGATGACAGAGTTTTGAGAATATATTTGTACCATATATTTAAAAAAAAAAAAAAAAAA
```

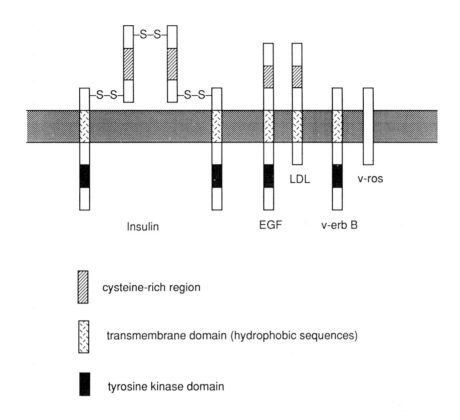

Fig. 5.5 — Schematic representation of the receptors for various agonists.

The EGF receptor actually has primary sequence homology with the insulin receptor. Unlike the insulin receptor, the EGF receptor is a single long polypeptide chain. It has two cysteine-rich regions and a tyrosine kinase activity. In fact, the tyrosine kinase activity provides the homology between the insulin receptor and the products of various oncogenes such as *v-erb-B*, *v-ros* and *v-fms*.

The most extensive sequence homology for the insulin receptor is with the receptor for IGF-1. Insulin and IGF-1 are very closely related and have a similar tertiary structure. Their receptors are also very similar, to the extent that each receptor shows a fair degree of affinity for the other hormone. The IGF-1 receptor is also a membrane glycoprotein consisting of two α- and two β-subunits of similar molecular weights to the insulin receptor: 135 000 and 90 000 respectively. The IGF-1 receptor α- and β-subunits are generated from a single precursor, and, like the insulin receptor, the IGF-1 receptor is a tyrosine protein kinase (see reviews by

◄ Fig. 5.4 — The insulin receptor cDNA sequence and the deduced amino acid sequence as reported by Ullrich *et al*. (1985). Black bar: putative transmembrane domain. Open bar: sites for *N*-glycosylation. Shading: cysteine residues. Boxes: precursor processing site. Reproduced by kind permission from Ullrich *et al*. (1985).

Rechler & Nissley, 1985; Duronio & Jacobs, 1988). The degree of glycosylation is similar and appears to be required for binding. Many generalizations have been made concerning the cross-reactivity of insulin and IGF-1 receptors. It is worth pointing out that in the vast majority of cases each hormone mediates its effects through its own receptor. It is generally thought that low concentrations of insulin act through the insulin receptor to cause a variety of metabolic events, such as stimulation of glucose transport, oxidation, etc. On the other hand, the growth-promoting effects of insulin tend to be ascribed to binding to IGF-1 receptors. The opposite appears the case with IGF-1 receptor, except that low concentrations of IGF-1 can have metabolic effects through its own receptor. In order to discriminate between these conflicting observations, Jacobs and colleages have developed a series of monoclonal antibodies to both insulin and IGF-1 receptors and the reader is referred to the review quoted above for more details of this work.

5.2 THE INSULIN RECEPTOR TYROSINE KINASE

Regulation of enzyme activity by reversible phosphorylation is a major mechanism for controlling the rate of metabolic pathways. Thus, many hormones exert their effects by altering the phosphorylation state of their target enzymes. The effects of insulin on such systems have been discussed in the previous chapter. Protein phosphorylation occurs mainly on serine or threonine residues, but over the last few years it has become apparent that phosphorylation also occurs at tyrosine residues, although it accounts for less than 0.05% of all protein phosphorylation on cells. Given this low level it has been suggested that the proteins that are phosphorylated at tyrosine residues must have a regulatory role. Several tyrosine kinases have been discovered and, interestingly, most appear to be encoded by oncogenes or growth-factor receptors. This observation has led to the suggestion that tyrosine kinase activity is exclusively concerned with the regulation of growth processes. Some of the growth-factor receptors that are known to posses a tyrosine kinase activity are IGF-1, EGF, PDGF, CSF, and, of course, insulin.

   In this section I review the evidence that the insulin receptor is a tyrosine kinase and discuss its possible physiological role. For general reviews on tyrosine kinases the reader is referred to Hunter & Cooper (1985) and Yarden & Ullrich (1988). Many reviews exist on the insulin receptor tyrosine kinase, but I would recommend those by Rosen (1987a,b), Goldfine (1987) and Van Obberghen & Gammeltoft (1987).

5.2.1 Phosphorylation of the insulin receptor

Phosphorylation of the insulin receptor was first demonstrated by Kasuga and co-workers (Kasuga et al., 1982a) in partially purified receptors. It has since been shown to occur in cell-free systems and in intact cells (Kasuga et al., 1982b,c; Avruch et al., 1982; van Obberghen & Kowalski, 1982). The phosphorylation of the receptor is increased about ten-fold upon insulin binding. It is a rapid, totally specific (no other agent will cause the phosphorylation), and dose-dependent phenomenon. The autophosphorylation of the insulin receptor has been reported to occur in many tissues and cell types.

The kinase activity of the insulin receptor is not a kinase that co-purifies with it but is intrinsic to the receptor. This has been shown by several observations. Thus, insulin receptors purified by WGA- and insulin-affinity chromatography show autophosphorylation in response to insulin. Further, insulin receptors immunoprecipitated with anti-insulin receptor antibodies are phosphorylated in response to insulin binding. It can therefore be inferred that the kinase activity resides within the receptor itself, since in these systems highly purified receptors were used.

Autophosphorylation of the insulin receptor occurs exclusively on the β-subunit. Moreover, the β-subunit also appears to exhibit the tyrosine kinase domain and the ATP-binding site. The latter has been shown by cross-linking studies using a photoaffinity ATP analogue, 8-azido-ATP (Roth & Cassell, 1983) or periodate-oxidized γ-^{32}-P-ATP (Van Obbergehen et al., 1983). Both compounds label the β-subunit alone. Further evidence supporting the localization of the tyrosine kinase to β-subunit comes from the sequence of the insulin receptor (Ullrich et al., 1985; Fig. 5.4). The cytoplasmic domain of the β-subunit has features corresponding to a kinase domain. Beginning at residue 991 this region has a sequence Gly-X-Gly-X-X-Gly, which is the consensus sequence for the ATP binding site for kinases (Hunter & Cooper, 1985). There is also a most important residue, Lys 1018, which attracts the negatively charged third phosphate of ATP and directs it to tyrosine residues.

The autophosphorylation of the insulin receptor is highly specific: only insulin will promote it. The kinase activity is independent of cAMP or Ca^{2+}, but, in cell-free systems, it appears to have a requirement for Mn^{2+} or Mg^{2+} at micromolar concentrations of ATP. The stimulation of autophosphorylation by insulin appears due to an increase in the V_{max} for ATP. In contrast, Mn^{2+} lowers the K_m for ATP. The kinase will only use ATP as the phosphate donor.

Autophosphorylation of the receptor occurs in several tyrosine residues. Of these, at least three residues have been proposed to be important for regulation. These include Tyr 960, 1150, 1316 and 1322. Site-directed mutagenesis experiments suggest that Tyr 1150 is essential for activity. When Tyr 1150 is changed to phenylalanine the ability of the receptor to autophosphorylate is decreased (Stadtmauer & Rosen, 1986a; Chou et al., 1987).

5.2.1.1 *Phosphorylation of the receptor in intact cells*
Insulin stimulates the phosphorylation of its receptor in intact cells as well as in purified preparations. A distinctive feature, however, is that in intact cells most of the phosphorylation occurs on serine and threonine residues, rather than tyrosine. In some cell types phosphorylation at tyrosine residues cannot be seen at all. However, when receptors from these cells are purified they can be phosphorylated at tyrosine residues (see, for example, Gazzano et al., 1983). The observation of serine phosphorylation has led to the suggestion that a serine kinase is associated with the receptor, and that serine phosphorylation acts as a negative-feedback regulator on the activity of the tyrosine kinase and hence of insulin action.

Various authors have tested this hypothesis by attempting to promote the serine phosphorylation of the insulin receptor through either a cAMP- or a protein kinase C-mediated mechanism. Thus, using purified systems protein kinase C phosphorylates the receptor β-subunit and this leads to a decrease in tyrosine kinase activity

(Bollag *et al.*, 1986). The same can be observed in intact cells. In Fao hepatoma cells, phorbol esters lead to activation of protein kinase C and phosphorylation of the insulin receptor on serine residues, which in turn results in a decreased tyrosine kinase activity (Takayama *et al.*, 1988). Similar results have been obtained when the phosphorylation of the tyrosine kinase is achieved in a cAMP-mediated way. Thus, increasing the cAMP content of cells leads to the phosphorylation of the insulin receptor at serine and threonine residues leading to a decrease in the tyrosine kinase activity of the receptor (Stadtmauer & Rosen, 1986b). Finally, it is worth pointing out that insulin has been reported to cause the tyrosine phosphorylation, and subsequent activation of a serine kinase (Yu *et al.*, 1987). Sale and colleagues have described two systems that characterize an insulin-sensitive serine kinase that can phosphorylate the receptor itself (Smith *et al.*, 1988). All these studies suggest that serine phosphorylation can indeed be considered a negative-feedback regulatory system for the insulin receptor tyrosine kinase activity.

An alternative way of regulating the phosphorylation of the insulin receptor in intact cells would be the activation of a specific phosphotyrosine phosphatase. No such phosphatase co-purifies with the receptor, although there is indeed a highly active tryosine-specific phosphatase in plasma membranes. Recently, a tyrosine phosphatase with activity towards the insulin receptor was purified (Strout *et al.*, 1988). A unique characteristic of this enzyme seemed to be its inhibition by Zn^{2+}. Little further information exists in this area.

5.2.2   Substrates for the insulin receptor tyrosine kinase

The discovery of the tyrosine kinase activity of the receptor has led to a search for putative substrates for the kinase. This question has been addressed by one of two methods. Many workers have tested the stimulation by insulin of tyrosine phosphorylation of a purified protein by the receptor tyrosine kinase. In other experiments, the putative substrates have been identified following incorporation of ^{32}P-inorganic phosphate ($^{32}P_i$) into cells and stimulation by insulin using SDS-PAGE, autoradiography and phosphoamino acid analysis. These methods have led to the identification of a variety of proteins that appear to be phosphorylated at tyrosine residues in response to insulin (Table 5.1).

In all cases the physiological importance of the proteins thus far found remains unknown. The proteins themselves are also unknown, being always identifed by their molecular weights on SDS-PAGE. The proteins that are phosphorylated in *in vitro* systems using purified receptor and protein do not have a known physiological role in insulin action either. Thus, in *in vitro* systems, insulin stimulates the tyrosine phosphorylation of casein, histone, angiotensin II, actin and various synthetic polypeptides containing tyrosine (e.g. Glu_4-Tyr). Some of these substrates, however, have been very useful in determining the activity of the receptor tyrosine kinase. The only protein shown to be phosphorylated at tyrosine residues in *in vitro* systems, and whose biological function could be of importance in insulin action, is calmodulin (Sacks & McDonald, 1988). Hoewever, this has not been shown *in situ*.

On interest too, are the guanine-nucleotide-binding proteins as possible substrates for the receptor tyrosine kinase. A guanine-nucleotide-binding protein has been proposed to be involved in the signal transduction of insulin receptors (see Chapter 6). It is thus interesting that G_i, G_o, transducin and ras can all be

Table 5.1 — Proteins phosphorylated at tyrosine residues in response to insulin

In vitro		In vivo	
Protein	Reference	Protein	Reference
Casein	Gazzano et al. (1983)	pp185 (a)	Kadowaki et al. (1987)
Histones	Gazzano et al. (1983)	pp185 (b)	Kadowaki et al. (1987)
Angiotensin I	Klein et al. (1985)	pp160	Yu et al. (1987)
Tyr-peptides	Zick et al. (1985)	pp120 (a)	Rees-Jones & Taylor (1985)
G_i and G_o	O'Brien et al. (1987)	pp120 (b)	Caro et al. (1987a)
Transducin	Zick et al. (1986)	pp116	Haring et al. (1987)
Lipocortins I and II	Karasik et al. (1988)	pp80	Kadowaki et al. (1987)
Calmodulin	Sacks & McDonald (1988)	pp46	Haring et al. (1987)
pp50	Kwok & Yip (1988)	pp15	Bernier et al. (1987)
pp35	Kwok & Yip (1988)	Lipocortin I	Karasik et al. (1988)

phosphorylated at tyrosine residues. It suggests the possibility that phosphorylation of a G protein may be a link between the receptor kinase and the target effector enzyme.

An interesting and novel *in vitro* method of searching for protein substrtates of the insulin receptor kinase has been presented by Kwok and Yip (1988). They used purified insulin receptors immobilized in resin by their binding to insulin–Sepharose. The immobilized receptor can be activated by autophosphorylation with ATP and then used to phosphorylate other proteins when they bind to the resin. Using this method they identified two liver proteins, unrelated to the insulin receptor, of 50 and 35 kDa that were specific substrates for the insulin receptor kinase and were not phosphorylated by other receptor kinases. Whilst the authors speculated as to the identity of these proteins, their function in unknown.

In intact cells, several proteins (see Table 5.1) whose molecular weight varies widely (from 15 000 to 185 000) have been shown to be possible substrates for the insulin receptor tyrosine kinase. Since none of these have been characterized or their function determined, I will just mention two whose role may be of importance to insulin action.

In an interesting study, Bernier and colleagues (1987) showed that insulin stimulated the tyrosine phosphorylation of a protein of 15 kDa (pp15) in intact 3T3-Li adippocyte cell line. Furthermore, pp15 accumulated when the cells were treated with phenylarsine oxide, an agent that inhibits insulin-stimulated glucose transport by complexing dithiols that are vicinal. Phosphorylation of pp15 and stimulation of glucose transport exhibited similar insulin dose–response curves. Their work thus suggested a possible role for pp15 in insulin signal transduction, but little else is known about this protein to date.

The lipocortins are also of interest. Lipocortins are a family of intracellular proteins that bind to phospholipids in the presence of calcium and inhibit phospholipase A_2 activity. Lipocortin I can be phosphorylated at tyrosine by the EGF receptor kinase, and lipocortin II by pp60src. Phosphorylation of lipocortins inhibits their activity (Powell & Glenney, 1987). In a recent study, Karasik et al. (1988) have shown both *in vitro* and in intact cells (hepatocytes) that lipocortin I can be phosphorylated at tyrosine residues in response to insulin. Lipocortin II can only be phosphorylated in an *in vitro* system. The role of lipocortin phosphorylation in insulin action, however, is totally unclear.

5.2.3 Physiological role of insulin receptor tyrosine kinase phosphorylation

The ultimate proof of whether a given reaction, protein, chemical, etc. is of importance to cell function is to show deficient functioning in its absence *in vivo*. There is therefore a central question that needs to be answered. Is the tyrosine kinase activity of the insulin receptor necessary for the metabolic effects of insulin to occur? The putative substrate for the tyrosine kinase is not directly relevant to the question; only whether the kinase activity itself is significant. Thus far, most evidence suggests that the answer to this question is yes. But before reviewing the evidence in favour of a physiological role for the tyrosine kinase, let me pose a problem. It is fair to argue that any pathway involved in mediating the action of insulin should be as sensitive to the hormone as the insulin-regulated metabolic pathway. Yet many workers have shown that the receptor kinase is quite insensitive to insulin, with half-maximal stimulation occurring at 2–10 nM insulin. This is in marked contrast to the effects of insulin on glucose uptake, glucose oxidation, lipolysis, and others, which, although variable between cell types, occur at concentrations at least two orders of magnitude smaller (20–100 pM). Although various arguments to explain this difference may be raised — e.g. the kinase effect may be amplified — it should, nevertheless, raise a doubt as to the physiological role of the tyrosine kinase activity of the insulin receptor.

Having posed this problem, I do however reiterate that most evidence suggests that the tyrosine kinase activity is a prerequisite for insulin action. The studies leading to this conclusion can be divided into three types. Firstly, the physiological role of the tyrosine kinase can be tested by checking whether there are defects in pathological conditions where the response to insulin is decreased, e.g. insulin-resistant conditions such as type II diabetes. Secondly, at the molecular level, it is possible to cause modifications in the kinase domain of the receptor and test if this alters the response to insulin. Finally, using antibodies against the receptor or the kinase, the relationship between them can be probed.

5.2.3.1 Studies on insulin resistance

In insulin-resistant hyperinsulinaemic obese mice, a decrease in insulin receptor tyrosine kinase has been shown in skeletal muscle (Le Marchand-Brustel *et al.*, 1985). In contrast, in a rat model of type II diabetes (neonatal administration of steptozotocin) no defect was observed in the liver (Kergoat *et al.*, 1988).

The most impressive studies in this area are those on NIDDM patients done by Caro and colleagues. These patients are insulin-resistant and no conclusive defect in the number of insulin receptors can be shown. Caro's group examined three groups of patients: normal control, obese non-diabetic and obese NIDDM. In both liver and adipose tissue they found marked decreases in receptor tryrosine kinase activity (Shinka *et al.*, 1987; Caro *et al.*, 1986). In muscle, the defect was less obvious as no differences were seen between obese NIDDM and obese non-diabetic patients, although there was a difference with normal controls (Caro *et al.*, 1987b). In view of the difference between muscle on the one hand and liver and adipose tissue on the other, it is difficult to speculate what the contribution of decreased receptor kinase activity to overall insulin resistance may be.

5.2.3.2   Site-directed mutagenesis studies

Studies in which the tyrosine kinase domain of the insulin receptor has been modified by site-directed mutagenesis have provided the strongest evidence for the absolute requirement of the receptor kinase activity for insulin action.

When mutant receptors containing phenylalanine instead of Tyr 1150 and Tyr 1151 are transferred into Chinese hamster ovary (CHO) cells, there is an inhibition of receptor autophosphorylation and a marked decrease in the sensitivity of these cells to insulin stimulation of 2-deoxyglucose uptake (Ellis *et al.*, 1986).

CHO cells expressing mutant receptors in which Lys 1018 at the ATP binding site has been replaced by alanine exhibit a markedly decreased sensitivity to insulin of various metabolic pathways including stimulation of glucose uptake, thymidine incorporation into DNA, S6 kinase activity and glycogen synthesis (Chou *et al.*, 1987; Ebina *et al.*, 1987).

Whilst these studies appear conclusive, a recent paper raises some interesting questions. White and colleagues have shown that mutation of Tyr 960 with phenyl-alanine has no effect on receptor autophosphorylation or on tyrosine kinase activity towards other substrates. However, in CHO cells transfected with this mutant, insulin signal transmission was inhibited (White *et al.*, 1988). These data suggest that autophosphorylation and receptor kinase activity are clearly not sufficient for insulin action.

5.2.3.3   Antibody studies

When monoclonal antibodies directed against the insulin receptor kinase domain of the β-subunit are microinjected into oocytes, insulin stimulation of cell maturation is inhibited (Morgan *et al.*, 1986). Furthermore, if these antibodies are introduced into mammalian cells (rat adipocytes or a human hepatoma cell line HepG2) they cause inhibition of tyrosine kinase activity and several metabolic processes regulated by insulin, including 2-deoxyglucose uptake, glycogen synthesis and ribosomal S6 protein phosphorylation (Morgan & Roth, 1987).

These data are supportive of a role for the receptor kinase in insulin action, but here as well there are conflictive studies. Thus, polyclonal antibodies directed to the α-subunit of the insulin receptor can stimulate glucose transport in adipocytes with no effect on the receptor kinase (Simpson and Hedo, 1984; Zick *et al.*, 1984).

The most interesting work in the antibody approach to studying the role of the receptor kinase is that of Goldfine and colleagues. These workers have used a panel of monoclonal antibodies directed against the α-subunit of the receptor. Two of these, MA-5 and MA-20, bind at a site distant from the insulin binding site, since insulin cannot displace the binding of the antibody to the receptor. On the other hand, the antibodies do inhibit insulin binding, which suggests that binding to the α-subunit may cause a conformational change within the subunit itself. These antibodies have the ability to stimulate glucose transport in adipocytes, but they do not stimulate the tyrosine kinase activity of the receptor. Thus, they do not lead to autophosphorylation of the receptor, nor to phosphorylation of exogenous substrates (Forsayeth *et al.*, 1987a,b). The antibodies are also able to stimulate glucose transport in cells transfected with receptor mutants in which the ATP binding site has been deleted.

The inference from these data is surprising for they contradict the established dogma. Namely, they suggest that autophosphorylation of the receptor and activation of the tyrosine kinase is not a prerequisite for insulin action. If the tyrosine kinase activity is not required for transmission of the signal, what is its role? It could be argued that autophosphorylation of the receptor is the result of a conformational change upon insulin binding, and that when the receptor is phosphorylated it is able to interact, or collide, with regulatory proteins, leading to transmission of the signal by means of second messengers or other such system. This scheme does not however agree with most of the evidence available, which does indeed support a physiological role for the kinase activity of the receptor.

5.3 INSULIN RECEPTOR INTERNALIZATION

Regulation of insulin receptor concentration at the plasma membrane is a complex process involving *de novo* synthesis and metabolism of the receptor. The first step in the metabolism of receptors is their internalization. Although these are important issues, little is known. A summary of current views follows.

Studies using radiolabelled or fluorescently labelled insulin have shown the internalization of the insulin receptor following the binding of insulin (Goldfine *et al.*, 1978; Schlessinger *et al.*, 1978). No agreement exists, however, on the subcellular localization of the internalized insulin receptor complexes. Insulin receptors have been shown to accumulate primarily in Golgi and Golgi-associated fractions, but also in endoplasmic reticulum, lysosome and the nuclear envelope. Localization of the insulin receptors in the Golgi lends support to the view that insulin receptors are recycled.

Internalization and recycling of receptors back to the membrane is a pathway common to proteins such as EGF, LDL, α-macroglobulin and asialoglycoproteins. The proteins undergo a receptor-mediated endocytosis where receptors are internalized at specific areas of the plasma membrane called 'coated pits'. The distinguishing feature of coated pits is that the cytoplasmic side is coated with the protein clathrin (for a review of 'coated pits' see Hopkins, 1985). Insulin receptors have indeed been shown to accumulate at such coated pits, following insulin binding (e.g. Fan *et al.*, 1982; Maxfield *et al.*, 1978). When the receptor enters the coated pit, vesicle formation ensues, resulting in a so-called 'endosome' or 'receptorsome'. These migrate to the lysome for degradation or can recycle back to the membrane by interacting with the Golgi (Fig. 5.6).

Insulin receptors have indeed been known to be recycled (Marshall *et al.*, 1981). In fact, internalization of insulin receptors may lead to the degradation of insulin, but not of the receptors. The presence of internalized receptors in lysosomes may just reflect the presence of internalized insulin and not the receptor, since most of these studies are done using radioactively labelled insulin. The acidic nature of the endosomal environment would be sufficient to remove the receptor from insulin itself.

Internalization of the insulin receptor seems to be an insulin-dependent process.

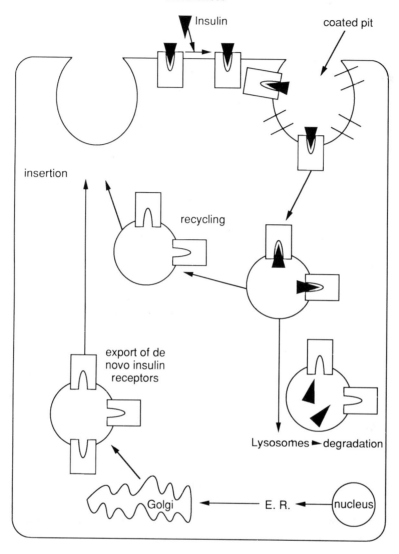

Fig. 5.6 — Recycling of insulin receptors.

On the other hand it is unclear what pathway is involved. Receptors can be recycled, degraded or retained undegraded for a certain period of time. The relative balance between all these states obviously regulates the amount of receptors at the membrane. Regulation of the total amount of receptor protein, however, cannot be accounted for by these processes alone and has to involve the regulation of gene expression.

REFERENCES

Avruch, J., Nemenoff, R. A., Blackshear, P. J., Pierce, M. W. & Osathanondh, R. (1982) *J. Biol. Chem.* **257**, 15 162–15 166.

Bernier, M., Laird, D. M. & Lane, M. D. (1987) *Proc. Nat. Acad. Sci.* **84**, 1844–1848.

Bollag, G. E., Roth, R. A., Beaudoin, J., Mochly-Rosen, D. & Koshland, D. E. J. (1986) *Proc. Nat. Acad. Sci.* **83**,5822–5824.

Caro, J. F., Ittoop, O., Paries, W. J., Meelheim, D., Flickinger, E. G., Thomas, F. Jenquin, M. & Silverman, J. F. (1986) *J. Clin. Invest.* **78**, 249–258.

Caro, J. F., Shafer, J. A., Taylor, S. I., Raju, S. M., Perrotti, N. & Shinka, M. K. (1987a) *Biochem. Biophys. Res. Comm.* **149**, 1008–1016.

Caro, J. F., Pories, W. F., Flickinger, E. G., Meelheim, D., Ittoop. O., Jenquin, M., Strinka, M. K. & Dohm, L. G. (1987b). *J. Clin. Invest.* **79**, 1330–1337.

Chou, C. K., Cull, T. J., Russell, D. S., Gherzi, R., Lebwohl, D., Ullrich, A. & Rosen, O. M. (1987) *J. Biol. Chem.* **262**, 1824–1847.

Cuatrecasas, P. (1972a) *Proc. Nat. Acad. Sci.* **69**, 1277–1287.

Cuatrecasas, P. (1972b) *Proc. Nat. Acad. Sci.* **69**, 318–322.

De Meyts, P., Gu, J. L., Shymko, R. M., Bell, G. & Whittaker, J. (1988) *Diabetologia* **31**, 484A.

Duronio, V. & Jacobs, S. (1988) In *Insulin receptors. Part B: Clinical assessment, biological response and comparison to the IGF-1 receptor.* Kahn, C. R., and Harrison, L. C. (Eds), Alan R. Liss, New York, pp. 3–18.

Ebina, Y., Ellis, L., Jarnagin, K., Edery, M., Graf, L., Clauser, E., Ou, J. H., Masiarz, F., Kan, Y. W. & Goldfine, I. D. (1985) *Cell* **40**, 747–758.

Ebina, Y., Arak, E., Taira, M., Shimada, F., Mori, M., Crank, C., Siddle, K. & Pierce, S. (1987) *Proc. Nat. Acad. Sci.* **84**, 704–708.

Ellis, L., Clauser, E., Morgan, D. O., Edery, M., Roth, R. A. & Rutter, W. J. (1986) *Cell* **45**, 721–732.

Fan, J. Y., Carpentier, J. L., Gordon, P., Van Obbergehen, E., Blackett, N. M., Grunfeld, C. & Orei, L. (1982) *Proc. Nat. Acad. Sci.* **79**, 7788–7791.

Forsayeth, J. R., Caro, J. F., Sinha, M. K., Maddux, B. A. & Goldfine, I. D. (1987a) *Proc. Natl. Acad. Sci. USA* **84**, 3448–3451.

Forsayeth, J. R., Montemurro, A., Maddux, B. A., DePirro, R. & Goldfine, I. D. (1987b) *J. Biol. Chem.* **262**, 4134–4140.

Fujita-Yamaguchi, Y., Choi, S., Sakamoto, Y. & Itakura, K. (1983) *J. Biol. Chem.* **258**, 5045–5049.

Fujita-Yamaguchi, Y. (1984) *J. Biol. Chem.* **259**, 1206–1211.

Gazzano, H., Kowalski, A., Fehlmann, M. & Van Obbergehen, E. (1983) *Biochem. J.* **216**, 575–582.

Goldfine, I. D. (1987) *Endocrine. Rev.* **8**, 235–255.

Goldfine, I. D., Jones, A. L., Hradek, G. T., Wang, K. Y. & Mooney, J. S. (1978) *Science* **202**, 760–763.

Haring, H. U., White, M. F., Machicao, F., Ermel, B., Schleicher, E. & Obermair, B. (1987) *Proc. Natl. Acad. Sci. USA* **84**, 113–117.

Hedo, J. A. (1988) In *Insulin Receptors. Part A: Methods for the study of structure and function.* Kahn, C. R. & Harrison, L. C. (Eds), Alan R. Liss, New York, pp. 83–100.

Hopkins, C. (1985) In 'Molecular Mechanisms of Transmembrane signalling'. Cohen, P. & Houslay, M. D. (Eds.), Elsevier, Amsterdam, pp 337–358.

Hunter, T. & Cooper, J. A. (1985) *Ann. Rev. Biochem.* **54**, 897–930.

Jacobs, S. & Cuatrecasas, P. (1981) *Endocrin. Rev.* **2**, 251–263.

Jacobs, S. & Cuatrecasas, P. (1985) *Ann. Rev. Pharmacol. Toxicol.* **23**, 461–479.

Jacobs, S., Hazum, E., Schechter, Y. & Cuatrecasas, P. (1979) *Proc. Nat. Acad. Sci.* **76**, 4918–4921.

Kadowaki, T., Koyasu, S., Nishida, E., Tobe, K., Izumi, T., Takaku, F., Sakai, H., Yahara, I. & Kasuga, M. (1987) *J. Biol. Chem.* **262**, 7342–7350.

Kahn, C. R. & Harrison, L. C. (1988) (Eds) *Insulin receptors. Parts A* and *B*, Alan R. Liss, New York.

Karasik, A., Pepinsky, R. B. Shallson, S. E. & Kahn, C. R. (1988) *J. Biol. Chem.* **263**, 11 862–11 867.

Kasuga, M., Karlsson, F. A. & Kahn, C. R. (1982a) *Science* **215**, 185–187.

Kasuga, M., Zich, Y., Blithe, D. L., Karlsson, F. A., Haring, H. V. & Kahn, C. R. (1982b) *J. Biol. Chem.* **257**, 9891–9894.

Kasuga, M., Hedo, J. A., Yamada, K. M. & Kahn, C. R. (1982c) *J. Biol. Chem.* **257**, 10 392–10 399.

Kergoat, M., Simon, J. & Portha, B. (1988) *Biochem. Biophys. Res. Comm.* **152**, 1005–1022.

Klein, H. H., Freidenberg, G. R., Cordera, R. & Olefski, J. M. (1985) *Biochem. Biophys. Res. Comm.* **127**, 254–263.

Kwok, Y. C. & Yip, C. C. (1988) *Biochem. J.* **248**, 27–33.

LeMarchand–Brustel, Y. L., Cremeaux, T., Balloti, R., & Van Obbergehen, E. (1985) *Nature* **315**, 676–679.

McClain, D. A., Henry, R. R., Ullrich, A. & Olefsky, J. M. (1988) *Diabetes* **37**, 1071–1076.

Marshall, S., Green, A. & Olefski, J. M. (1981) *J. Biol. Chem.* **256**, 11 464–11 470.

Massague, J. & Czech, M. P. (1982) *J. Biol. Chem.* **257**, 6729–6738.

Maxfield, F. R., Schlessinger, J., Schlechter, Y., Paston, I. C. & Wittingham, M. C. (1978) *Cell* **14**, 805–810.

Morgan, D. O., Ho, L., Korn, L. J. & Roth, R. A. (1986) *Proc. Nat. Acad. Sci.* **83**, 328–332.

Morgan, D. O. & Roth, R. A. (1987) *Proc. Nat. Acad. Sci.* **84**, 41–45.

O'Brien, R. M., Houslay, M. D., Milligan, G. & Siddle, K. (1987) *FEBS Lett.* **212**, 281–288.

Pressin, J. E., Mottola, C., Yu, K.-T. & Czech, M. P. (1985) Subunit structure and regulation of the insulin–receptor complex. In *Molecular basis of insulin action*, Czech, M. P. (Ed.), Plenum Press, New York, pp. 3–29.

Pilch, P. F. & Czech, M. P. (1979) *J. Biol. Chem.* **254**, 3375–3381.

Powell, M. A. & Glenney, J. E. (1987) *Biochem. J.* **247**, 321–328.

Rechler, M. M. & Nissley, S. P. (1985) *Ann. Rev. Physiol.* **47**, 425–442.

Rees-Jones, R. W. & Taylor, S. I. (1985) *J. Biol. Chem.* **260**, 4461–4467.

Rosen, O. (1987a) *Science* **237**, 1452–1458.

Rosen, O. (1987b) *Harvey Lect.* **82**, 105–122.

Roth, R. A. & Cassell, D. J. (1983) *Science* **219**, 299–301.

Sacks, D. B. & McDonald, J. M. (1988) *J. Biol. Chem.* **263**, 2377–2383.

Schlessinger, J. Y., Schlechter, Y., Wittingham, M. C. & Paston, I. (1978) *Proc. Nat. Acad. Sci.* **75**, 2659–2663.

Shinka, M. K., Pories, W. J., Flickinger, E. G., Meelheim, D. & Caro, J. F. (1987) *Diabetes* **36**, 620–625.

Simpson, I. A. & Hedo, J. A. (1984) *Science* **223**, 1301–1304.

Smith, D. M., King, M. J. & Sale, G. J. (1988) *Biochem. J.* **250**, 509–519.

Stadtmauer, L. & Rosen, O. M. (1986a) *J. Biol. Chem.* **261**, 10 000–10 005.

Stadtmauer, L. & Rosen, O. M. (1986b) *J. Biol. Chem.* **261**, 3402–3407.

Strout, H. V., Vicario, P. P., Saperstein, R. & Slater, E. E. (1988) *Biochem. Biophys. Res. Comm.* **151**, 633–640.

Takayama, S., White, M. & Kahn, C. R. (1988) *J. Biol. Chem.* **263**, 3440–3447.

Ullrich, A., Bell, J. R., Chen, E. Y., Herrera, R., Petruzzelli, L. M., Dull, T. J., Gray, A., Coussens, L., Liao, Y. C., Tsubokawa, M., Seeburg, P. H., Grunfeld, C., Rosen, O. M. & Ramachandran, J. (1985) *Nature* **313**, 756–761.

White, M. F., Livingston, J. N., Backer, J. M., Lauris, V., Dull, T. J., Ullrich, A. & Kahn, C. R. (1988) *Cell* **54**, 641–649.

Van Obberghen, E. & Gammeltoft, S. (1987) *Experientia (Suppl.)* **53**, 31–45.

Van Obberghen, E. & Kowalski, A. (1982) *FEBS Lett.* **143**, 179–182.

Van Obberghen, E., Rossi, B., Kowalski, A., Gazzano, H. & Ponzio, G. (1983) *Proc. Natl. Acad. Sci. USA* **80**, 945–949.

Yarden, Y. & Ullrich, A. (1988) *Ann. Rev. Biochem.* **57**, 443–478.

Yip, C. C. (1988) In *Insulin receptors. Part A*, Kahn, C. R. & Harrison, L. C. (Eds), Alan R. Liss, New York, pp. 101–110.

Yip, C. C., Hsu, H., Patel, R. G., Hawley, D. M., Maddux, B. A. & Goldfine, I. D. (1988) *Biochem. Biophys. Res. Comm.* **157**, 321–329.

Yu, K. L., Khalaf, N. & Czech, M. P. (1987) *Proc. Natl. Acad. Sci. USA* **84**, 3972–3976.

Zick, Y., Rees-Jones, R. W., Taylor, S. I., Gorden, P. & Roth, J. (1984) *J. Biol. Chem.* **259**, 4396–4400.

Zick, Y., Grunberger, G., Rees-Jones, R. W. & Comi, R. (1985) *Eur. J. Biochem.* **148**, 177–182.

Zick, Y., Sagi-Eisenberg, R., Pines, M., Gierschik, P. & Spiegel, A. M. (1986) *Proc. Natl. Acad. Sci. USA* **83**, 9294–9297.

6

Molecular mechanisms of insulin signal transduction

Hormones and other extracellular stimuli that act via cell-surface receptors require a system or mechanism to translate their binding to the receptor into a cellular response. These mechanisms are generally referred to as transmembrane signalling systems, and usually involve the generation of small molecules within the cell that lead to the various cellular changes. These small molecules are referred to as second messengers. The basic components of a transmembrane signalling system are therefore a receptor coupled to the generation of a second messenger. There are however a few intervening steps as follows. The vast majority of receptors studied to date appear to be coupled to guanine-nucleotide regulatory proteins (G proteins). These in turn are coupled to the so-called effector enzyme, which is the one responsible for the generation of a second messenger. Once the messenger is generated it then acts upon its target enzymes, thereby causing the cellular responses. The terminology used in this area is usually similar to that of electronics and thus the coupling regulatory proteins are occasionally referred to as the 'transducers' and the effector enzyme as the 'amplifier'.

To date, two signalling systems have been well described and characterized. Moreover, with the exception of insulin, they account for the transmembrane signalling systems employed by most extracellular stimuli studied. Lately, a third second-messenger system that appears to be involved mainly, or exclusively, with the actions of insulin has been described. There exist hundreds of reviews or books that describe the first two signalling systems. The main point of this chapter is to describe research in the area of second messengers as it pertains to insulin, and therefore only brief summary descriptions of each of the main two signalling systems are given.

The idea that insulin has a second messenger has been prevalent in the literature probably since the discovery of cAMP as a second messenger for adrenalin. In fact the existence of a second messenger for insulin continues to be one of the most controversial issues surrounding the mechanism of action of this hormone. As discussed in a review by Denton and colleagues in 1981 on this topic, the number of substances that have been proposed as second messengers for insulin is high (Denton *et al.*, 1981). The list includes cAMP, cGMP, Ca^{2+}, H_2O_2, changes in pH, changes in membrane potentials, and a few more esoteric candidates. Recently, however, a novel class of inositol phospholipids has been proposed to be the precursor for an inositol-containing second messenger for insulin. These are the topics discussed in the present chapter.

6.1 THE cAMP SYSTEM

Of all the second messenger systems studied, the one involving the generation of cAMP must be the best known and characterized. The number of agonists that act via changes in the concentration of cAMP is too large to list. So is the number of cellular processes evoked by cAMP. The characterization of the system goes back to the discovery by Sutherland and Rall of cAMP itself. The enzymatic system responsible for its synthesis (adenylate cyclase produces cAMP from ATP) and its breakdown (cAMP phosphodiesterase will produce AMP from cAMP), was soon characterized. Many studies have also described the mechanisms by which cAMP elicits its actions; namely, the activation of cAMP-dependent protein kinase (occasionally referred to as protein kinase A). The system is well-described in many excellent reviews including those by Ross & Gilman (1980), Gilman (1984, 1987), Birnbaumer *et al.* (1985). A brief summary of the current views on this system follows.

The receptors that affect cAMP formation can be classified into two types: R_s receptors, which stimulate adenylate cyclase and hence cause elevation of cAMP levels; and R_i receptors, which inhibit adenylate cyclase and hence decrease the levels of cAMP. There are many receptors under each category, but typical examples of R_s receptors include the β_1 and β_2 adrenergic receptors, and receptors for glucagon, ACTH, etc.; and for R_i α_2-adrenergic receptors, and receptors for opioids, adenosine (in adipose tissue), and others. The means by which these receptors are coupled to adenylate cyclase is through the G proteins G_s and G_i (see Fig. 6.1).

The involvement of a G protein in signal transduction was first suggested by the studies of Rodbell and colleagues (Rodbell *et al.*, 1971) who showed a requirement for GTP in the activation of adenylate cyclase. Many advances have followed since then including the purification of various G proteins and the isolation of cDNAs for some of them. G proteins are a family of guanine(GTP)-binding proteins whose function is to couple receptors to their effector enzymes. The best characterized G proteins are G_s and G_i and a G protein that couples light-activated rhodopsin to cGMP phosphodiesterase, called transducin or G_t. Other G proteins have been proposed to couple certain receptors to other messenger systems, or suggested from primary sequence homologies, including G_o, G_p, and ras, the product of the cellular oncogene *c-ras*.

G_s, G_i, and G_t consist of three subunits (α, β, γ) of different molecular weights. Interestingly, the β-subunit(35 kDa) appears to be the same for all three G proteins, but the three α-subunits are very different ($G_s\alpha$, 46 kDa; $G_i\alpha$, 41 kDa; $G_t\alpha$, 40 kDa) and contain the GTP binding site. The γ-subunit is around 8 kDa; this subunit also appears common to all G proteins.

The biological mechanism by which G proteins act appears to be as follows.

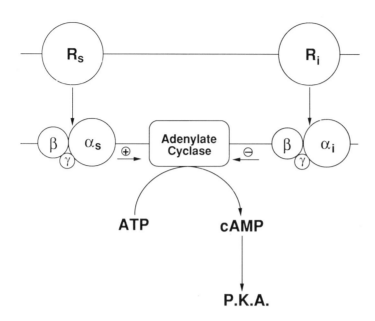

Fig. 6.1 — Schematic representation for receptors regulating cAMP levels.

Hormone binding to its receptor causes a conformational change that results in the release of an activated α-subunit from the complex. The free α-subunit interacts with and activates (or inhibits) the effector enzyme. It should be pointed out that the above mechanism is believed to occur for G_s and G_t. The mechanism by which G_i inhibits adenylate cyclase is still unclear. It could either be via direct interaction, as suggested above, or by the release of β-subunits from G_i following the dissociation of $G_i\alpha$. The free β-subunits could then bind to $G_s\alpha$ subunits, thus preventing any possible acivation. In all three regulatory proteins the β-subunit deactivates the free α-subunit by recombining with it. This results in the hydrolysis of GTP to GDP, and therefore it means that the β-subunit is stimulating a GTPase activity inherent in the α-subunit. A cycle of active and interactive states therefore exists between associated and dissociated forms of the α- and β-subunits. The reader is referred to the reviews by Gilman for details.

Much of the evidence leading to the involvement of G proteins in receptor signal transduction has been obtained using either cholera toxin or pertussis toxin. These toxins promote the NAD^+-dependent ADP-ribosylation of the α-subunits. This covalent modification results in the inhibition of the receptor-stimulated GTPase activity of the G protein. The mechanism via which this is achieved is different in each case. Cholera toxin causes the dissociation and permanent activation of $G_s\alpha$, whereas pertussis toxin acts on $G_i\alpha$, preventing its dissociation and hence blocking its inhibition. Therefore both toxins promote increases in cAMP levels. These toxins have been used as a criteria for the existence of G proteins in any given receptor system, as will be discussed in relation to insulin below.

6.1.1 Effects of insulin on the cAMP system

Some of the cellular effects of insulin can be ascribed to lowering the concentration of cAMP. This is particularly relevant in the liver, where insulin opposes the action of glucagon, or in adipose tissue, where there is antagonism between insulin and adrenalin. In contrast, in skeletal muscle, most of insulin's actions are direct effects upon a given metabolic pathway. In the liver insulin will only decrease cAMP levels once they have been elevated by glucagon, but not when insulin is presented alone. The regulation of cAMP levels through the relationship between glucagon and insulin is highly complex and has been the focus of research of many groups, particularly that of Houslay and colleagues. The reader is referred to several reviews of their work for full details (Houslay 1984, 1985).

Insulin can decrease cellular cAMP levels by activating cAMP phosphodiesterase activity, as first reported by Loten & Sneyd (1970). The effect can be observed in both liver and adipose tissue 'particulate' fractions. Several forms of cAMP phospho-diesterase exist in cells (see e.g. Heyworth *et al.*, 1983). At least two types of cAMP phosphodiesterase are generally described in liver and adipose tissue, namely the 'low K_m' and 'high K_m' variants. In liver there appear to be as many as eight different enzymes but insulin seems to activate only the 'low K_m' type(s). The recent work of Houslay's group has been concerned with the identification of the particular species of insulin-sensitive phosphodiesterases. Insulin appears to cause the activation of at least three different cAMP phosphodiesterases in liver, all of which are of the 'low K_m' type. They differ in their cellular location as well as in other characteristics.

The first of the insulin-stimulated hepatic phosphodiesterases is a peripheral enzyme that is associated with the plasma membrane by apparent ionic interactions with integral membrane proteins. It has been purified to homogeneity and shown to be a monomer of 52 kDa. The enzyme exhibits unusual kinetic behaviour and shows activation at low substrate concentrations following the activation by insulin (March-mont & Houslay, 1980a,b; Marchmont *et al.* 1981; Housley & Marchmont, 1981).

Insulin also activates a so-called 'dense-vesicle' phosphodiesterase, believed to be the phosphodiesterase described in many studies in adipocytes or hepatocytes. It has also been purified and shown to be a dimer of two 57-kDa subunits (Pyne *et al.*, 1987). An unusual property of this enzyme is its ability to be activated by glucagon as well as insulin. It is difficult to reconcile a true physiological role for this enzyme in the action of insulin with its activation by glucagon also (Wallace *et al.*, 1984).

A third phosphodiesterase is also activated by insulin in intact hepatocytes (Wilson *et al.*, 1983). This activation is not seen in homogenates or plasma membrane fractions, as is the case with the other two enzymes. Houslay (1986) suggests that this may be the enzyme whose activity may be modulated by a second messenger directly. Indeed, some very recent studies of theirs have shown the presence of a putative mediator in hepatocytes, capable of activating the enzyme (Pyne & Houslay, 1988). For details of the purifaction and characteristics of the insulin-sensitive cAMP phosphodiesterases, the reader is referred to a recent review by Houslay and co-workers (Houslay *et al.*, 1988).

Two unusual features of the insulin activation of the peripheral cAMP phospho-diesterase are the insulin-stimulated cAMP-dependent phosphorylation of the phosphodiesterase and the further activation of the enzyme by GTP (Heyworth *et al.*, 1983). This last observation led Houslay and colleagues to propose the existence of an insulin-receptor-linked G protein, which they called G_{ins} (Houslay & Heyworth, 1983). The evidence that these authors have provided over recent years in favour of this hypothesis is varied, but I will attempt to summarize its distinctive features.

Glucagon can block the effects of insulin on cAMP phosphodiesterase activation and adenylate cyclase inhibition. These effects occur simultaneously, and at the same concentrations as the glucagon-induced desensitization of its own effects on adenylate cyclase (see Houslay, 1985, for details). The desensitization appears to involve an inhibition or uncoupling of G_s, and hence it would seem plausible that the inhibition by glucagon of insulin's effects would be due to an uncoupling, or inhibition, of a G protein specifically associated with insulin. The specificity is necessary as activation of G_s does not activate the phosphodiesterase. Likewise, the effect of insulin cannot be related to G_i since pertussis toxin does not block it. However, pertussis toxin does block the inhibition by insulin of adenylate cyclase, an effect suggesting that insulin's effects could be mediated via G_i. In a very elegant study, Houslay and co-workers provided a response to this problem. Streptozotocin- or alloxan-induced diabetes in rats causes a decrease of about 90% in the levels of G_i in liver plasma membranes. In these circumstances, insulin treatment of plasma membranes does not cause inhibition of adenylate cyclase. However, if the animals are treated with metformin, the ability of insulin to inhibit adenylate cyclase is restored, in spite of no accompanying changes in the levels of G_i. These data clearly suggest that insulin's inhibition of adenylate cyclase in liver is not due to G_i but probably due to some other specific G protein (Gawler et al., 1988).

Two other pieces of evidence suggest the existence of a putative G_{ins}. Insulin can inhibit the cholera-toxin-induced ADP-ribosylation of a protein of 25 kDa in liver plasma membranes, suggesting this protein as a possible candidate for the α-subunit of G_{ins} (Heyworth et al., 1985). Finally, insulin has been shown to cause the activation of a GTPase activity in human platelets (Gawler & Houslay, 1987). Both of these data would be typical behaviour of a functioning G protein. G_{ins} remains to be isolated, characterized and purified. When this is accomplished, its role in insulin action will be more easily tested.

In summary, some of the effects of insulin, particularly those in liver, can be associated with a modulation of cAMP levels. This means that insulin, in some way, is affecting the cAMP signalling system. A possible site of its action are the G proteins that regulate the activation and inhibition of adenylate cyclase. A candidate G protein has been proposed that is specific for insulin but its identity has, to date, not been forthcoming.

6.2 THE INOSITOLTRISPHOSPHATE—DIACYLGLYCEROL SYSTEM

The second major receptor-activated transmembrane signalling system is one whose elucidation goes back to the work of Hokin and Hokin in the early 1950s (Hokin & Hokin, 1953). In this system, various agonists can activate a phospholipase C which hydrolyses phosphatidylinositol 4,5-bisphosphate (PtdIns4,5P$_2$) to yield inositol 1,4,5-trisphosphate (Ins1,4,5P$_3$) and sn-1,2-diacylglycerol (DG), both of which act as second messengers (Fig. 6.2). There have been a multitude of reviews on this topic in recent years. I would recommend those by Downes & Mitchell (1985), Hokin

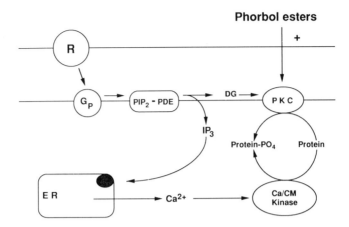

Fig. 6.2 — Coupling for calcium-mobilizing receptors.

(1985), Nishizuka (1986), and Berridge (1984, 1987). A discussion on this topic could be very lengthy since it could cover the evidence for a receptor-mediated system on the one hand, and the details of inositol metabolism on the other. Considerable detail on both can be found in the reviews listed above. For the purposes of this chapter, however, it is necessary to discuss, briefly, some details on the metabolism of inositol phosphates and their respective lipids, since they are of relevance regarding the next section discussing the role of glycosylphosphatidylinositols in insulin action.

6.2.1 Inositol lipid metabolism

Phosphatidylinositol (PtdIns) constitutes only a few per cent of membrane phospho-lipids; its phosphorylated derivatives phosphatidylinositol-4-phosphate (PtdIns4P) and PtdIns4,5P$_2$, constitute only a few per cent of inositol lipids in cells. PtdIns can be sequentially phosphorylated by two kinases to yield PtdIns4P and PtdIns4,5P$_2$ (Fig. 6.3). Two phosphatases exist that can dephosphorylate the two derivatives back to PtdIns.

PtdIns4,5P$_2$ is the substrate for the generation of the second messenger Ins1,4,5P$_3$. The other two inositol lipids have also been suggested to be used by certain agonists (see Berridge, 1987, for discussion), but this does not seem to form part of a transmembrane signalling system. In order for PtdIns4,5P$_2$ to generate Ins1,4,5P$_3$ it has to be hydrolysed by a specific phospholipase C. Many stimuli have now been shown to stimulate the hydrolysis of PtdIns4,5P$_2$, and this now appears a rather ubiquitous mechanism of signal transduction (lists of the agonists acting through this system can be found in the reviews listed above).

As is the case with any second-messenger system, a mechanism must exist for its generation and for its breakdown, otherwise cells would be in a permanently activated state. In the case of Ins1,4,5P$_3$, breakdown occurs by a series of sequential dephosphorylations that result in Ins1,4P$_2$, Ins1P (and Ins4P), and finally, inositol (Fig. 6.4). The phosphatases involved have different degrees of specificity. Thus,

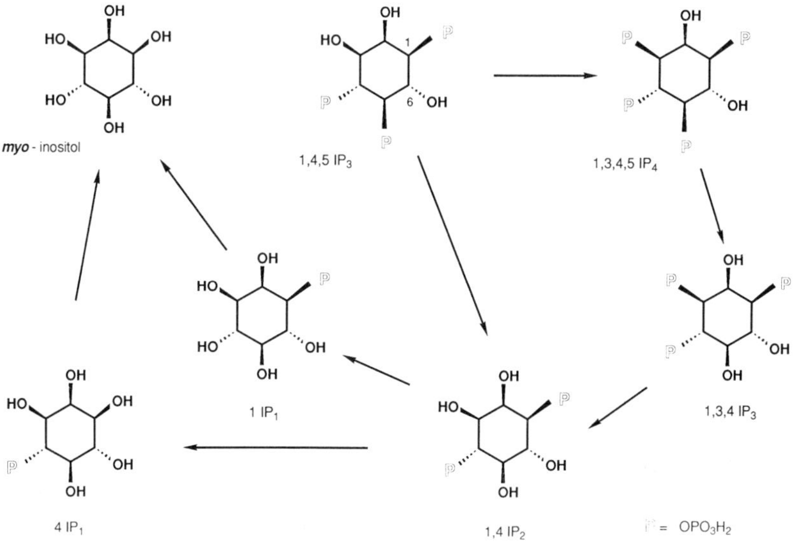

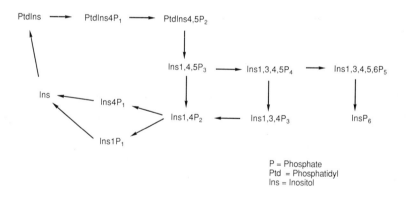

Fig. 6.3 — Metabolism of inositol phosphates.

Fig. 6.4 — Metabolic cycle of the inositol phosphates.

$Ins1,4,5P_3$-5-phosphatase is very specific towards the position of the phosphate in the inositol ring (Storey *et al.*, 1984). The enzyme is insensitive to lithium, unlike other inositol phosphatases, but can be inhibited by spermine and by 2,3-diphosphoglycerate, (Seyfred *et al.*, 1984). Dephosphorylation of $Ins1,4P_2$ is accomplished by an enzyme not showing any degree of specificity towards the phosphate groups as both Ins1P and Ins4P can be produced.

Phospholipase C can also produce inositol 1 : 2 cyclic 4,5-trisphosphate (cIns1 : 2,4,5P$_3$) as well as Ins1,4,5P$_3$ (Ishii *et al.*, 1986). The breakdown of this compound follows a similar route of dephosphorylation as Ins1,4,5P$_3$.

In recent years a new route of breakdown of Ins1,4,5P$_3$ has been discovered. This pathway also results in inositol derivatives phosphorylated at further hydroxyl groups (see Fig. 6.4). Ins1,4,5P$_3$ can be phosphorylated by a specific kinase to yield inositol 1,3,4,5-tetrakisphosphate (Ins1,3,4,5P$_4$) (Irvine *et al.*, 1986). Ins1,3,4,5P$_4$ can then be dephosphorylated to inositol 1,3,4-triphosphate (Ins1,3,4P$_3$). Ins1,3,4,5P$_4$ can also be the precursor for InsP$_5$ and InsP$_6$, compounds that have recently been suggested to have a messenger role (Vallejo *et al.*, 1987).

A characteristic common to many inositolphosphate phosphatases is their inhibition by Li$^+$, which has been utilized in the methods to isolate the inositolpolyphosphates. Thus cells can be incubated in the presence of Li$^+$, so as to be able subsequently to separate chromatographically the various inositol derivatives.

6.2.2 Mechanism of second-messenger action

The most distinctive feature of the inositol messenger system is its bifurcating nature. Thus, two messengers are generated upon the agonist-stimulated phospholipase C hydrolysis of PtdIns4,5,6P$_2$: Ins1,4,5P$_3$ and DG. Therefore, two mechanisms of activation of cellular processes are called upon simultaneously. The system is versatile and sensitive.

Each of the arms of the bifurcating signal has to be broken down so as to avoid constant activation. I have discussed above the metabolism of inositol lipids. The breakdown of DG follows routes that have been known for a long time in fatty acid metabolism. DG can be metabolized by its phosphorylation to phosphatidic acid by DG kinase or its hydrolysis to monoacylglycerol by DG lipase. Monoacylglycerol can then be further hydrolysed to produce arachidonic acid, which can served as a precursor in eicosanoid production.

The mechanisms whereby Ins1,4,5P$_3$ and DG lead to cellular events such as proliferation are distinct, if somehow interacting. The DG generated at the plasma membrane acts by activating protein kinase C (Nishizuka, 1984, 1986). Protein kinase C requires calcium and phosphatidylserine (PS) for activation. The effects of calcium and DG on the enzyme appear synergistic. Activation of protein kinase C involves a translocation of the enzyme to the plasma membrane, a process that may need calcium. When activated, protein kinase C can then phosphorylate its various target enzymes. A peculiar feature of this system is that the intracellular targets for phosprylation by protein kinase C that are physiologically relevant are still uncharacterized. Nevertheless, the involvement of protein kinase C in processes that involve cell replication, proliferation, and suchlike is reasonably well-documented. A review of protein kinase C is well beyond the scope of this section and the reader is referred to the reviews by Nishizuka quoted above.

Ins1,4,5P$_3$ operates via a completely different mechanism. Hydrolysis of PtdIns4,5P$_2$ appears to be exclusive to agonists that operate by mobilization of calcium. Cellular calcium mobilization can occur from extracellular and intracellular sources. In Chapter 2, while discussing the process of insulin secretion, I described two phases involved in this process, and that they appeared to correlate with the mobilization of calcium from intracellular sites and with the entry of calcium from outside the cell. This seems to be a generalized system of elevating cytosolic calcium concentrations, and thus applicable to many, if not all, of the calcium-mobilizing receptors. It is in these processes that $Ins1,4,5P_3$ is intimately involved. $Ins1,4,5P_3$ causes the release of calcium from the endoplasmic reticulum, thereby increasing cytosolic calcium concentration. This function has been demonstrated for a multitide of receptors in different cell types (see Berridge, 1987) and whilst it is of obvious significance in receptor-mediated systems, Berridge suggests that it could even have a role in modulating basal calcium concentrations through small changes in inositol lipid metabolism. The mobilization of calcium from the endoplasmic reticulum in response to $Ins1,4,5P_3$ does not appear to be mediated through a pump mechanism, but more likely results from a channel-type process.

It now seems clear that the mechanism by which $Ins1,4,5P_3$ causes calcium mobilization is through its binding to a specific receptor in the endoplasmic reticulum. Specific binding sites for $Ins1,4,5P_3$ have been located in the microsomal fraction of adrenal cortex and liver (Spat *et al.*, 1986a,b). Binding of radiolabelled $Ins1,4,5P_3$ can be displaced by other inositol phosphates, but the presence of phosphate groups at the 4 and 5 positions aplpears essential. Affinity probes of $Ins1,4,5P_3$ have been produced (Hirata *et al.*, 1985) and it is only a question of time till the receptor is fully purified and characterized.

6.2.3 Summary of the hypothesis

The $Ins1,4,5P_3$/DG signalling system is a unique bifurcating method of transmitting signals to the inside of the cell. In the majority of cases examined, the two arms of this signal are synergistic. The hypothesis proposes that upon ligand binding to its receptor a phospholipase C is activated, which causes the hydrolysis of $PtdIns4,5P_2$ to yield $Ins1,4,5P_3$ and DG. DG activates protein kinase C and the latter causes changes in protein phosphorylation. $Ins1,5P_3$ causes mobilization of calcium from the endoplasmic reticulum and hence activates calcium-stimulated processes. A good example of this signalling system was presented in Chapter 2 during the discussion on the mechanism of insulin secretion. Is this signalling system involved, however, in the action of insulin?

6.2.4 Insulin action and the $Ins1,4,5P_3$/DG system

In the last few years there has been considerable interest in the effects of insulin on inositol lipid metabolism. Some of this is related to the possibility that some of the effects of insulin could be due to alterations in the $Ins1,4,5P_3$/DG pathway. Others have examined the putative involvement of inositol glycolipids in insulin action. The latter is discussed in the next section. Here I shall concentrate on the role of changes in PtdIns and its derivatives in the action of insulin.

Insulin has been reported to cause an increase in the synthesis and/or levels of inositol phospholipids in adipose tissue and BC3H1 myocytes (Farese *et al.*, 1982, 1984, 1985a,b, 1987; Cooper *et al.*, 1987). Thus, insulin causes an increase in ^3H-inositol labelling of PtdIns, PtdIns4P and $PtdIns4,5P_2$, suggesting an increase in synthesis. Additionally, insulin has been shown to cause an increase in the level or labelling of DG and phosphatidic acid (PA) (Farese *et al.*, 1984, 1985a, 1987; Saltiel *et al.*, 1986, 1987). Furthermore, insulin has been reported to increase the activity of protein kinase C (Cooper *et al.*, 1987). This latter observation is of significance since some of the actions of insulin have been suggested to be mediated in part by an increase in the activity of protein kinase C. The evidence for this is indirect, as it relies heavily on the fact that phorbol esters (which activate protein kinase C) can have insulin-mimetic activity in various cells with respect to glucose transport and the patterns of phosphorylation of target proteins (see Chapter 4) (Blackshear *et al.*, 1985; Farese *et al.*, 1985b; Kirsch *et al.*, 1985; Chu & Granner, 1986). Finally, treatment of cells with phospholipase C has been reported to cause insulin-like effects, such as stimulation of pyruvate dehydrogenase (Koepfer-Hobelsberger & Wieland, 1984) or lipogenesis (Saltiel & Sorbara-Cazan, 1987).

All these data do not seem to converge into a single mechanism for insulin's effects on inositol lipid metabolism. Thus, both synthesis (the effects on PtdIns lipids, DG and PA) and breakdown (the effects on protein kinase C and those of phospholipase C) of inositol lipids appear to be invoked in the action of insulin. The various reports are therefore, somewhat contradictory. In a study designed to clarify these issues Augert & Exton (1987) examined the metabolism of inositol lipids in adipose tissue in response to insulin and oxytocin was chosen because of its insulin-like effects in adipose tissue (Hanif *et al.* 1982a,b). Their study revealed that while oxytocin caused the breakdown of polyphosphoinositides to yield DG and inositol phosphates, insulin did not do so. Therefore, they suggested that the insulin-like effects of oxytocin were not due to the breakdown of PtdIns or its phosphorylated derivatives. However, their study confirmed previous observations that insulin stimulated the incorporation of ^{3}H-inositol into PtdIns, PtdIns4P and PtdIns4,5P$_2$, as well as that of ^{3}H-glycerol into these lipids and also PA, phosphatidylserine and phosphatidylethanolamine. Their study is worth mentioning here for having addressed the controversy surrounding the effects of insulin on inositol lipid metabolism. They suggested that the effects of insulin on these systems are to increase the activity of one or more enzymes involved in the biosynthesis of PA from glycerol or glycerol 3-phosphate.

In a recent study, Farese and colleagues (Farese *et al.*, 1988a) support the observations of Augert & Exton (1987) with respect to the lack of effect of insulin on phospholipase C breakdown of inositol lipids. They suggest that insulin stimulates the *de novo* synthesis of PA and DG, as well as causing a breakdown of phosphatidylethanolamine (PE) and/or phosphatidylcholine (PC). A signalling system involving PC has been proposed even though no agonists have been shown to operate exclusively or partially through it (Besterman *et al.*, 1986).

6.3   THE INVOLVEMENT OF GLYCOSYLPHOSPHATIDYLINOSITOL (GPI) IN INSULIN ACTION

For many years a search for a second messenger for insulin has been underway. Insulin is the one hormone for which no clear second messenger system has been shown to exist. Many compounds have been proposed to be such a messenger (or 'mediator', according to the terminology used in this area) and over the years changes in cyclic nucleotide content, hydrogen peroxide, changes in pH, changes in polyphosphoinositides or even internalization of insulin itself have been suggested to mediate the action of the hormone (see Denton *et al.*, 1981, for review). The search has generated controversy at various times, and it is fair to say that even today there are more critics than advocates for even the most promising of second messengers.

One of the problems in this area is the pleiotropic nature of insulin's cellular effects. As discussed in previous chapters, insulin elicits responses in many different systems, from glucose transport to DNA synthesis. These effects also differ in the time at which they occur. These characteristics have made the choice of a test system for searching for an insulin second messenger rather difficult. Most workers in this field have used target enzymes whose activity is altered by insulin in the short term.

In the late 1970s, at least three groups (those of Larner, Jarret and Czech) reported the generation of a compound or compounds in response to insulin that was able to modulate the activities of intracellular enzymes such as glycogen synthase (Larner et al., 1979; Jarett & Seals, 1979; Seals & Czech, 1980). The compounds in question were purported to be small peptides that were generated by insulin activation of a plasma membrane protease. The peptides were suggested to cause the activation of kinases and/or phosphatases. The existence of more than one peptide was reconciled with the different mechanisms involved in the activation by insulin of target enzymes. Thus, one peptide would activate kinases, leading to protein phosphorylation, while another peptide would activate phosphatases leading to dephosphorylation (see the reviews on this area by Jarett & Kiechle, 1984; Jarett et al., 1982; Larner et al., 1982). This theory, like so many others in the 'mediator' field, had too much hypothesis and too little solid evidence. The 'peptide mediators' were never completely purified, characterized or sequenced, and in fact, over the following few years the theory seemed to disappear from the literature.

Other authors had also reported various substances purported to be 'mediators' of insulin action. Thus, Saltiel and co-workers reported the generation of a 'mediator(s)' capable of modulating the activities of cAMP phosphodiesterase, adenylate cyclase, pyruvate dehydrogenase and acetyl CoA carboxylase (Saltiel et al., 1981, 1982, 1983). These compounds appeared to contain inositol, but none of the known inositol phosphates could cause similar effects. The work at the time on glycosyl-phosphatidylinositol (GPI) anchors of proteins led to the realization that these structures could serve as precursors for the insulin 'mediator'. Thus, in 1986 Saltiel and Cuatrecasas reported that insulin caused the cleavage of a GPI to generate an inositol phosphoglycan (IPG) and diacylglycerol.

6.3.1   Anchoring of membrane proteins by GPIs

Before discussing in detail the current hypothesis on the role of GPIs in insulin action, some background information on the role of these inositol lipids in the attachment of proteins to the plasma membrane is required. For detailed reviews on this topic see Ferguson & Williams (1988) and Low & Saltiel (1988).

A specific role of PtdIns in the anchoring of proteins to the plasma membrane was first shown for alkaline phosphatase (Low & Zilversmit, 1980). The original, and subsequent, studies showed that various proteins could be released from the plasma membrane by treatment of cells with specific phosphatidylinositol phospholipase C (PI-PLC) (purified from bacterial soruces). The detection of covalently attached myo-inositol to acetylcholinesterase from the electric organ of Torpedo (Futerman et al., 1985) and alkaline phosphatase from human placenta (Low et al., 1987) confirmed the hypothesis that several proteins were attached to the plasma membrane of cells through a phosphatidylinositol anchor.

The use of purified bacterial PI-PLC has allowed the discovery of many proteins anchored in this manner (Table 6.1). The list of proteins includes hydrolytic enzymes, cellular antigens, cell adhesion molecules, complement regulatory protein, and the coat protein of *Trypanosoma brucei*. Thus, there is no functional homology between any of these proteins. There also appears to be no primary sequence homology between them. In fact, it is unclear what directs a protein to be anchored in the manner as opposed to any other mechanism of membrane attachment. Some of the clues to this puzzle have come from looking at the sequence of the mature protein and comparing them to the sequence that would be derived from their respective cDNAs. When this is done, these proteins show a C-terminal segment present in the cDNA but absent in the mature protein. There are no homologies between these segments, except that they are all highly hydrophobic. The reader is referred to the review by Ferguson & Williams (1988) for a discussion of this topic.

Current knowledge of the structure of GPI is based on the details of the structure for the GPI of the variant surface glycoprotein of *T. brucei*, a protein that coats the protozoan's surface. The only other GPI whose structure is known in detail is that of rat brain Thy-1 antigen, which differs only slightly from that of *T. brucei* (see Ferguson *et al.*, 1988; Homans *et al.*, 1988). Fig. 6.5 summarizes the essential feature of GPIs. The protein's C-terminal amino acid is amide linked through its α-carboxyl group to ethanolamine. The ethanolamine group is linked to the 6-hydroxyl group of mannose through a phosphodiester bond. The mannose is part of a glycan structure, which contains several hexoses and ends in glucosamine. The glucosamine in GPIs is non-N-acetylated, a feature that serves as a diagnostic for these structures, since it rarely occurs in most biological systems. Moreover, the presence of a free amino group allows the structure to be selectively cleaved by nitrous acid. Finally, the glucosamine is glycosidically linked through its C-1 position to the 6-hydroxyl group of the inositol ring in PtdIns. The two GPIs whose structures are known in detail show conservation of a core glycan structure consisting of $(Mann)_3GlcNH_2$ attached to PtdIns.

The presence of ethanolamine, glucosamine and *myo*-inositol has been confirmed for most of the proteins analysed in detail so far. In some proteins, a second ethanolamine is also found, and this has been confirmed in the structure of the GPI anchor for Thy-1 (Homans *et al.*, 1988). The presence of *chiro*-inositol, an unusual inositol isomer, has been shown in at least three cases (see Low & Saltiel, 1988, for details). Interestingly, *chiro*-inositol has been shown to be present in the GPI precursor for the insulin 'mediator' (Mato *et al.*, 1987b).

An unusual modification to the structure of GPIs has been found in the anchor of acetylcholinesterase from human erythrocytes. While the enzyme from bovine erythrocytes can be completely released from the membrane by treatment with PI-PLC, the human enzyme appears to be resistant to enzyme cleavage. Recent detailed studies by Rosenberry and colleagues have shown that the reason for this is palmitylation of the inositol molecule at the 2-hydroxyl (Roberts *et al.*, 1987, 1988a,b). Since the major product of PI-PLC hydrolysis is 1,2-cyclic inositol phosphate, palmitylation at C-2 does not allow enzymic cleavage.

The cellular or physiological role of GPI anchors is unclear. Various suggestions have been made, but few have been conclusively demonstrated. The presence of a GPI anchor is believed to confer some unique characteristics on the protein. The protein may now become more mobile in the membrane bilayer (see Ferguson &

Table 6.1 — Cell surface proteins with a glycosyl-phosphatidylinositol membrane anchor (adapted from Ferguson & Williams (1988) and Low & Saltiel (1988))

Protein

Hydrolytic enzymes
  Alkaline phosphatase
  5′-Nucleotidase
  Acetylcholinesterase
  Alkaline phosphodiesterase
  Trehalase
  p63 protease (*Leishmania major*)
  Renal dipeptidase
  Merozoite protease (*Plasmodium falciparum*)

Mammalian antigens
  Thy-1
  RT-6 (rat lymphoctes)
  T-cell activating protein and other Ly-6 antigens
  Qa
  Carcinoembryonic antigen
  Blast-1 (human lymphocytes)
  CD-14 (human monocytes)

Cell adhesion
  Neural cell adhesion molecule (N-CAM)
  Heparan sulphate proteoglycan
  LFA-3 (human lymphocytes)
  Contact site A (*Dictyostelium discoideum*)

Protozoal coat proteins and antigens
  Variant surface glycoprotein (*Trypanosoma brucei*)
  Surface proteins (*Paramecium primaurella*)
  Ssp-4 (*T. cruzi*)
  Tegument protein (*Schistosoma mansoni*)

Miscellaneous
  Decay accelerating factor
  130-kDa hepatoma glycoprotein
  34-kDa placental growth factor
  Scrapie prion protein
  PH-20 protein (guinea pig sperm)
  GP-2 (pancreatic zymogen granule)

Williams, 1988, for discussion), even though the advantage of such a characteristic is not immediately obvious. The presence of a GPI will confer upon the protein the ability to be rapidly released by phospholipase cleavage. Agonists such as hormones

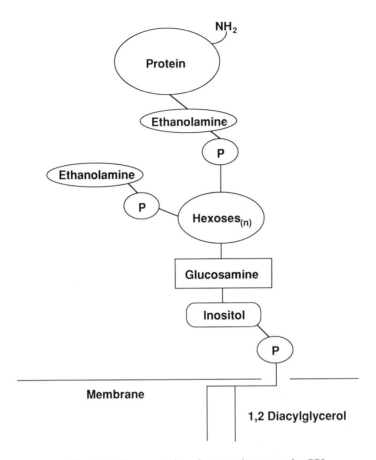

Fig. 6.5 — Representation of a general structure for GPIs.

could cause the cleavage of GPI-anchored proteins as part of their normal cellular actions. Indeed, it has been shown that insulin can cause the release of lipoprotein lipase (Chan *et al.*, 1988) and heparan sulphate proteoglycan (Ishihara *et al.*, 1987). The fact that several of the GPI-anchored proteins are cellular antigens may go towards supporting a role for GPI-anchorage to be involved in cell–cell communication.

6.3.2   GPI in insulin action
The first evidence that led Saltiel and colleagues to the conclusion that the insulin 'mediator(s)' were products of GPI cleavage come from their experiments with PI-PLC. They were able to show that both insulin and PI-PLC could release from liver plasma membrane two compounds with insulin-like activity (Saltiel & Cuatrecasas, 1986). In the BC3H1 myocyte cell line, metabolic prelabelling showed that the lipid precursor and its products could be labelled with inositol and glucosamine, which confirmed a possible homology with GPI anchors (Saltiel *et al.*, 1986).

Based on these observations, Saltiel and colleagues proposed that insulin caused the activation of a PI-PLC which cleaved a GPI precursor to yield IPGs that mediated some of the actions of the hormone, such as activation of cAMP phosphodiesterase (Saltiel *et al.*, 1986; Saltiel & Cuatrecasas, 1986).

6.3.2.1   Structure of the insulin-sensitive GPI

Since the original study by Saltiel and colleagues, other workers have repeated similar kind of experiments. Their data and those of Saltiel show that these compounds can be metabolically labelled with inositol, glucosamine, phosphate, and saturated fatty acids (Saltiel *et al.*, 1986, 1987; Mato *et al.*, 1987a). While Saltiel has reported labelling with myristic acid (Saltiel *et al.*, 1987), Mato *et al.* (1987a) found no such labelling in H35 hepatoma cells but instead could label the liquid precursor with palmitic acid.

One of the constant criticisms levelled against this hypothesis is the apparent failure to propose a concrete structure for these compounds. Indeed, to date, the type of analysis that has been performed on GPI anchors (see Ferguson *et al.*, 1988; Homans *et al.*, 1988) has not been done on the insulin-sensitive GPI or its products (IPGs). The only attempts to such a characterization have been those of Mato and his colleagues on the one hand and Larner and colleagues on the other. Mato and co-workers purified the lipid from H35 hepatoma cells and from rat liver, and performed analysis of neutral sugars and inositol as alditol acetates, and analysed the inositol as the trimethylsilyl ethers. Their data suggested that the insulin-sensitive GPI contains a phosphatidyl-*chiro*-inositol glycosidically linked to a non-*N*-acetylated glucosamine, which in turn is linked to three or four galactoses. The presence of a total of three phosphate residues was also reported (Mato *et al.*, 1987b). In contrast, Larner and co-workers reported that the lipid contains galactosamine (Larner *et al.*, 1988).

In a review of this area, Saltiel & Cuatrecasas (1988) have speculated on the existence of a phosphodiester bond between two hexoses (see Fig. 6.6) with the IPG

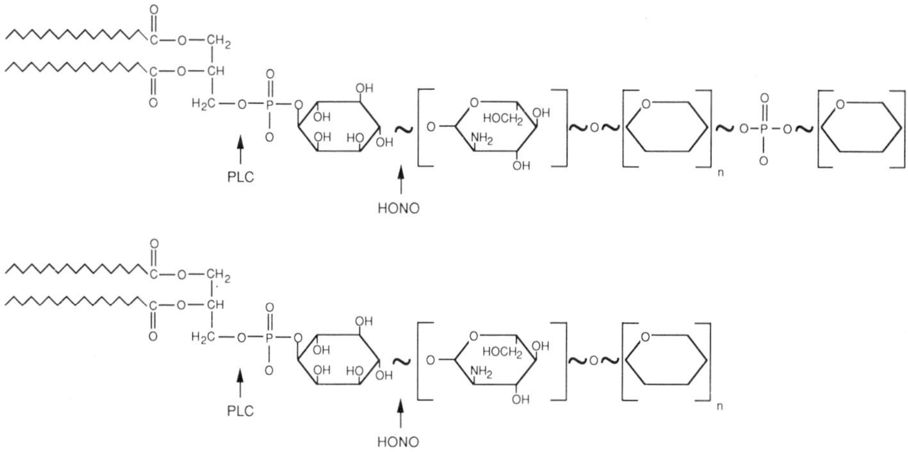

Fig. 6.6 — Possible structures of IPGs.

containing a total of four sugars. The evidence for this structure has not been forthcoming.

It must be said that quite clearly there is a lot of variability in proposed structures. Even for someone involved in this area of research, it is difficult to determine if the differences are due to experimental procedures, tissue sources, or any other possibilities. The one comment to make about these 'mediators' is that, contrary to other previous candidates, these structures, or rather structures of this type, have been confirmed to be biologically active by different groups, and that some sort of consensus has begun to emerge in the literature.

6.3.2.2 Biological activities of IPGs

The polar head groups of the insulin-sensitive GPIs have been shown to have a multitude of biological effects in different systems. Thus, the phospho-oligosaccharide (in Mato's terminology) can mimic the effects of insulin to promote protein phosphorylation/dephosphorylation (Alemany et al., 1987), inhibit lipolysis (Kelly et al., 1987) and stimulate lipogenesis (Saltiel & Sorbara-Cazan, 1987) in intact adipocytes. The 'mediator' also mimics the effects of insulin on cAMP phosphodiesterase (Saltiel & Cuatrecasas, 1986), adenylate cyclase (Saltiel, 1987), pyruvate kinase, glycogen phosphorylase and cAMP levels (Alvarez et al., 1987). However, the one insulin-like effect that these compounds do not appear to have is stimulation of glucose transport (Kelly et al., 1987).

An oligosaccharide produced from the conditioned medium of Reuber hepatoma cells has been reported to be labelled with glucosamine and to exhibit similar characteristics to those of the IPGs described by Saltiel, Mato, Jarett or Larner (Witters & Watts, 1988). This compound has been shown to cause activation of acetyl CoA carboxylase, DNA synthesis, and the phosphorylation of two proteins which are also phosphorylated in response to insulin (Witters et al., 1988). Like the IPGs discussed above, it failed to stimulate glucose transport, as well as amino acid transport.

The mechanism by which the 'mediator' or IPG causes its effects is unclear, but a possible clue might have been provided by the work of Villalba et al. (1988) who showed that the oligosaccharide could inhibit the activity of cAMP-dependent protein kinase without either altering the binding of cAMP to the protein or competing with ATP for binding.

It is of great interest that the IPG or 'mediator' is capable of eliciting biological responses in intact cells when its proposed structure predicts a highly charged compound, and, thus, one unlikely to cross the plasma membrane. In this context, it is important to note that the effect of the 'mediator' has been reported to be blocked by incubation with inositolmonophosphate, suggesting the existence of a receptor or transporter system that takes up the compound into the cell (Saltiel & Sorbara-Cazan, 1987). The experiments of Ishihara et al. (1987) also proposed a similar kind of inositolphosphate-mediated transport system. No evidence exists to date for any such systems.

6.3.2.3 Cellular and other considerations

Since the GPI anchors of proteins are located at the outer layer of the plasma membrane, the location of the insulin-sensitive GPI has been a topic of controversy.

From a logical perspective, any second messenger precursor should be located on the inner layer of the plasma membrane; the example being PtdIns4,5P$_2$. However, the evidence for the insulin-sensitive GPI is poor. According to Larner and his colleagues, insulin actually cleaves a GPI protein anchor (Romero *et al.*, 1988) instead of a free lipid, as proposed by Saltiel (see Saltiel & Cuatrecasas, 1988; Low & Saltiel, 1988).

An interesting method for addressing this issue has been used by Mato and co-workers. They have attempted to radiolabel the free amino group of glucosamine to determine the relative location of the lipid. The GPI was reacted with the imidoester [1-^{14}C]-isethionyl acetimidate, which, in addition to labelling GPIs, labels phosphatidylethanolamine and phosphatidylserine. They find that most of the insulin-sensitive GPI is located at the outer layer of the plasma membrane (Alvarez *et al.*, 1988). The authors suggested that a paracrine mode of action exists with respect to the 'mediator'. If this is confirmed it would represent a somewhat bizarre signalling system, whereby the 'mediator' lies outside the cell and has to enter it to exert its biological actions. It is not clear whether this hypothesis is realistic or not. Amongst the more recent developments in this area are the reports of generation of antibodies to the insulin-sensitive GPI (Whatmore *et al.*, 1988). The antibodies show the disappearance of the GPI from tissues following short exposure to insulin. Recently, a similar GPI has been proposed to be involed in the action of EGF, IGF-1 and ACTH (Farese *et al.*, 1988b,c).

Unfortunately, in spite of the relatively large consensus on the role of GPIs in insulin action, more questions than answers exist. Controversy has always surrounded the area of second messengers for insulin and probably always will, at least until such time as a clear chemical structure exists and pathways for its synthesis and breakdown in the short term are proposed.

REFERENCES

Alemany, S., Mato, J. M. & Stralfors, P. (1987) *Nature* **330**, 77–79.

Alvarez, J. F., Cabello, M. A., Feliu, J. E., & Mato, J. M. (1987) *Biochem. Biophys. Res. Commun.* **147**, 765–771.

Alvarez, J. F., Varela, I., Ruiz-Albusac, J. M. & Mato, J. M. (1988) *Biochem. Biophys. Res. Commun.* **152**, 1455–1462.

Augert, G. & Exton, J. (1987) *J. Biol. Chem.* **263**, 3600–3609.

Berridge, M. J. (1984) *Biochem. J.* **220**, 345–360.

Berridge, M. J. (1987) *Ann. Rev. Biochem.* **56**, 159–193.

Besterman, J. M., Duronio, V. & Cuatrecasas, P. (1986) *Proc. Natl. Acad. Sci. USA* **83**, 6785–6789.

Birnbaumer, J., Codina, J. Mattera, R., Cerione, R. A., Hildebrandt, J. D., Sunyer, T., Rojas, F. J., Caron, M. G., Lefkowitz, R. J. & Iyengar, R. (1985) In *Molecular mechanisms of transmembrane signalling*, Cohen, P. & Houslay, M. D. (Eds), Elsevier, Amsterdam, pp. 131–178.

Blackshear, P. J., Witters, L. A., Girard, P. R., Juo, J. F. & Quamo, S. N. (1985) *J. Biol. Chem.* **260**, 13 304–13 315.

Chan, B. L., Lisanti, M. P., Rodriguez-Boulan, E. & Saltiel, A. R. (1988) *Science* **241**, 1670–1672.

Chu, D. T. W. & Granner, D. K. (1986) *J. Biol. Chem.* **261**, 16848–16853.

Cooper, D., Konda, T. S., Standaert, M. L., Davis, J. S., Pollet, R. J. & Farese, R. V. (1987) *J. Biol. Chem.* **262**, 3633–3639.

Denton, R. M., Brownsey, R. W. & Belsham, G. J. (1981) *Diabetologia* **21**, 347–363.

Downes, C. P. & Michell, R. H. (1985) In *Molecular mechanisms of transmembrane signalling*, Cohen, P. & Houslay, M. D. (Eds), Elsevier, Amsterdam, pp. 3–56.

Farese, R. V., Larson, R. E. & Sabir, M. A. (1982) *J. Biol. Chem.* **257**, 4042–4045.

Farese, R. V., Barnes, D. E., Davis, J. S., Standaert, M. L. & Pollet, R. J. (1984) *J. Biol. Chem.* **259**, 7094–7100.

Farese, R. V., Davis, J. S., Barnes, D. E., Standaert, M. L., Babischkin, J. S., Hock, R., Rosic, N. K. & Pollet, R. J. (1985a) *Biochem. J.* **231**, 269–278.

Farese, R. V., Standaert, M. L., Barnes, D. E., Davis, J. S. & Pollet, R. J. (1985b) *Endocrinology* **116**, 2650–2653.

Farese, R. V., Konda, T. S., Davis, J. S., Standaert, M. L. & Pollet, R. J. (1987) *Science* **238**, 586–589.

Farese, R. V., Cooper, D. R., Konda, T. S., Nair, G., Standaert, M. L., Davis, J. S. & Pollet, R. J. (1988a) *Biochem. J.* **256**, 175–184.

Farese, R. V., Cooper, D. R., Konda, T. S., Nair, G., Standaert, M. L. & Pollet, R. J. (1988b) *Biochem. J.* **256**, 185–188.

Farese, R. V., Nair, G., Standaert, M. L. & Cooper, D. R. (1988c) *Biochem. Biophys. Res. Commun.* **156**, 1346–1352.

Ferguson, M. A. J. & Williams, A. F. (1988) *Ann. Rev. Biochem.* **57**, 285–320.

Ferguson, M. A. J., Homans, S. W., Dwek, R. A. & Rademacher, T. W. (1988) *Science* **239**, 753–759.

Futerman, A. H., Low, M. G., Ackerman, K. E., Sherman, W. L. & Silman, I. (1985) *Biochem. Biophys. Res. Commun.* **129**, 312–317.

Gawler, D. & Houslay, M. D. (1987) *FEBS Lett.* **216**, 94–98.

Gawler, D., Milligan, G. & Houslay, M. D. (1988) *Biochem. J.* **249**, 537–542.

Gilman, A. G. (1984) *Cell* **36**, 577–579.

Gilman, A. G. (1987) *Ann. Rev. Biochem.* **56**, 615–649.

Hanif, K., Goren, H. J., Hollenberg, M. D. & Lederis, K. (1982a) *Mol. Pharmacol.* **22**, 381–388.

Hanif, K., Goren, H. J., Hollenberg, M. D. & Lederis, K. (1982b) *Can. J. Physiol. Pharmacol.* **60**, 993–997.

Heyworth, C. M., Wallace, A. V. & Houslay, M. D. (1983) *Biochem. J.* **214**, 99–110.

Heyworth, C. M., Whetton, A. D., Wong, S., Martin, B. R. & Houslay, M. D. (1985) *Biochem. J.*, **228**, 593–603.

Hirata, M., Kukita, M., Sasaguri, T., Suematsu, E., Hashimoto, T. & Koga, T. (1985) *J. Biochem.* **97**, 1575–1582.

Hokin, L. E. (1985) *Ann. Rev. Biochem.* **54**, 205–235.

Hokin, M. R. & Hokin, L. E. (1953) *J. Biol. Chem.* **203**, 967–977.

Homans, S. W., Ferguson, M. A. J., Dwek, R. A., Rademacher, T. W., Anand, R. & Williams, A. F. (1988) *Nature* **333**, 269–272.

Houslay, M. D. (1984) *Trends Biochem. Sci.* **9**, 39–40.

Houslay, M. D. (1985) In *Molecular mechanisms of transmembrane signalling*, Cohen, P. & Houslay, M. D. (Eds), Elsevier, Amsterdam, pp. 279–334.

Houslay, M. D. (1986) *Biochem. Soc. Trans.* **14**, 183–193.

Houslay, M. D. & Heyworth, C. M. (1983) *Trends Biochem. Sci.* **8**, 449–452.

Houslay, M. D. & Marchmont, R. J. (1981) *Biochem. J.* **198**, 703–706.

Houslay, M. D., Pyne, N. J. & Cooper, M. E. (1988) *Method Enzymol.* **159**, 751–760.

Irvine, R. F., Letcher, A. J., Heslop, J. P. & Berridge, M. J. (1986) *Nature* **320**, 631–634.

Ishihara, M., Fedarko, N. S. & Conrad, H. E. (1987) *J. Biol. Chem.* **262**, 4708–4716.

Ishii, H., Connolly, T. M., Bross, T. E. & Majerus, P. W. (1986) *Proc. Natl. Acad. Sci. USA* **83**, 6397–6401.

Jarett, L. & Seals, J. R. (1979) *Science* **206**, 1407–1408.

Jarett, L., Kiechle, F. L. & Parker, J. C. (1982) *Fed. Proc.* **41**, 2736–2741.

Jarett, L. & Kiechle, F. L. (1984) Vitamins & Hormones **41**, 51–78.

Kelly, K. L., Merida, I., Wong, E. H. A., DiCenzo, D. & Mato, J. M. (1987) *J. Biol. Chem.* **262**, 15285–15290.

Kirsch, D., Obermaier, B., & Haring, H. U. (1985) *Biochem. Biophys. Res. Commun.* **128**, 824–832.

Koepfler-Hobelsberger, B. & Wieland, O. H. (1984) *Mol. Cell. Endocr.* **36**, 123–129.

Larner, J., Galasko, G., Cheng, K., DePaoli-Roach, A. A., Huang, I., Daggy, P. & Kellog, J. (1979) *Science* **206**, 1408–1410.

Larner, J., Cheng, K., Schwartz, C., Kirkuchi, K., Tamura, S., Creacy, S., Dubler, R., Galasko, G., Pullin, C. & Katz, M. (1982) *Fed. Proc.* **41**, 2724–2729.

Larner, J., Huang, L. C., Schwartz, C. F., Oswald, A. S., Shen, T. Y., Kinter, M., Tang, G. Z. & Zeller, K. (1988) *Biochem. Biophys. Res. Commun.* **151**, 1416–1426.

Loten, E. G. & Sneyd, J. G. T. (1970) *Biochem. J.* **120**, 187–193.

Low, M. G. & Saltiel, A. R. (1988) *Science* **239**, 268–275.

Low, M. G. & Zilversmit, D. B. (1980) *Biochemistry* **19**, 3913–3918.

Low, M. G., Futerman, A. H., Ackerman, K. E., Sherman, W. R. & Silman, I. (1987) *Biochem. J.*, **241**, 615–619.

Marchmont, R. J. & Houslay, M. D. (1980a) *Nature* **286**, 904–906.

Marchmont, R. J. & Houslay, M. D. (1980b) *Biochem. Soc. Trans.* **8**, 537–538.

Marchmont, R. J., Ayad, S. & Houslay, M. D. (1981) *Biochem. J.* **195**, 645–652.

Mato, J. M., Kelly, K. L., Abler, A. & Jarett, L. (1987a) *J. Biol. Chem.* **262**, 2131–2137.

Mato, J. M., Kelly, K. L., Abler, A., Jarett, L., Cashel, J. A. & Zopf, D. (1987b) Biochem. Biophys. Res. Commun. **146**, 764–770.

Nishizuka, Y. (1984) *Nature* **308**, 693–698.

Nishizuka, Y. (1986) *Science* **233**, 305–312.

Pyne, N. J. & Houslay, M. D. (1988) *Biochem. Biophys. Res. Commun.* **156**, 290–296.

Pyne, N. J., Cooper, M. E. & Houslay, M. D. (1987) *Biochem. J.* **242**, 33–42.

Roberts, W. L., Kim, B. H. & Rosenberry, T. L. (1987) *Proc. Natl. Sci. USA* **84**, 7817–7821.

Roberts, W. L., Myher, J. J., Kuksis, A., Low, M. G. & Rosenberry, T. L. (1988a) *J. Biol. Chem.* **263**, 18766–18775.

Roberts, W. L., Santikarn, S., Reinhold, V. N. & Rosenberry, T. L. (1988b) *J. Biol. Chem.* **263**, 18776–18784.

Rodbell, M., Birnbaumer, L., Pohl, S. L. & Krans, H. M. J. (1971) *J. Biol. Chem.* **246**, 1877–1882.

Romero, G., Luttrell, L., Rogol, A., Zeller, K., Hewlett, E. & Larner, J. *Science* **240**, 509–511.

Ross, E. & Gilman, A. G. (1980) *Ann. Rev. Biochem.* **49**, 533–564.

Saltiel, A. R. (1987) *Endocrinology* **120**, 967–972.

Saltiel, A. R. & Cuatrecasas, P. (1986) *Proc. Natl. Acad. Sci. USA* **83**, 5793–5797.

Saltiel, A. R. & Cuatrecasas, P. (1988) *Am. J. Physiol.* **255**, C1–C11.

Saltiel, A. R. & Sorbara-Cazan, L. R. (1987) *Biochem. Biophys. Res. Commun.* **149**, 1084–1092.

Saltiel, A. R., Jacobs, S., Siegel, M. & Cuatrecasas, P. (1981) *Biochem. Biophys. Res. Commun.* **102**, 1041–1047.

Saltiel, A. R., Siegel, M., Jacobs, S. & Cuatrecasas, P. (1982) *Proc. Natl. Acad. Sci. USA* **79**, 3513–3517.

Saltiel, A. R., Doble, A., Jacobs, S. & Cuatrecasas, P. (1983) *Biochem. Biophys. Res. Commun.* **110**, 789–795.

Saltiel, A. R., Fox, J. A., Sherline, P. & Cuatrecasas, P. (1986) *Science* **233**, 967–972.

Saltiel, A. R., Sherline, P. & Fox, J. A. (1987) *J. Biol. Chem.* **262**, 1116–1121.

Seals, J. R. & Czech, M. P. (1980) *J. Biol. Chem.* **255**, 6529–6531.

Seyfred, M. A., Farrell, L. E., Wells, W. W. (1984) *J. Biol. Chem.* **259**, 13 204–13 208.

Spat, A., Bradford, P. G., McKinney, J. S., Rubin, R. P. & Putney, J. W. (1986a) *Nature* **319**, 514–516.

Spat, A., Fabiato, A. & Rubin, R. P. (1986b) *Biochem. J.* **233**, 929–932.

Storey, D. J., Shears, S. B., Kirk, C. J. & Michell, R. H. (1984) *Nature* **312**, 374–376.

Vallejo, M., Jackson, T., Lightman, S. & Hardy, M. R. (1987) *Nature* **330**, 656–658.

Villalba, M., Kelly, K. L. & Mato, J. M. (1988) *Biochim. Biophys. Acta* **968**, 69–70.

Wallace, A. V., Heyworth, C. M. & Houslay, M. D. (1984) *Biochem. J.* **222**, 177–182.

Whatmore, A. J., Spitalnik, S. L., Gaulton, G. N. & Jarett, L. (1988) *Arch. Biochem. Biophys.* **264**, 355–360.

Wilson, S. R., Wallace, A. V. & Houslay, M. D. (1983) *Biochem. J.* **216**, 245–248.

Witters, L. A. & Watts, T. D. (1988) *J. Biol. Chem.* **263**, 8027–8036.

Witters, L. A., Watts, T. D., Gould, G. W., Lienhard, G. E. & Gibbs, E. M. (1988) *Biochem. Biophys. Res. Commun.* **153**, 992–998.

7

Summary and perspectives

7.1 SUMMARY

Nearly two years ago, I wrote a short review article on the mechanism of action of insulin for the *Nature* (Espinal, 1987). Few things have changed since then, but what follows is an updated version of that article.

Insulin exerts a central physiological role in the regulation of numerous processes. The magnitude of its importance can be measured by the magnitude of the disease that its absence or inability to function causes. For anyone unsure of this, looking at the consequences of diabetes would assure them otherwise. The effects of insulin occur over a range of times and in many different tissues. At the molecular level, however, some common patterns emerge. Thus, most of the enzymes whose activity is modified by insulin are dephosphorylated in response to the hormone. A few exceptions exist, and indeed some proteins are phosphorylated, but the physiological relevance in these cases has not been demonstrated as yet.

In spite of the amount of knowledge we have about insulin, even now, more than sixty years after its discovery, the mechanism of action of this hormone continues to be a puzzle. Most hormones and other agonists need to bind to specific cell surface receptors in order to exert their cellular effects. This is the first required step in a long cascade of events. Indeed this is the case with insulin. The insulin receptor belongs to the tyrosine kinase family of cell surface receptors. The kinase is activated upon binding of insulin to its receptor and leads to the autophosphorylation of the receptor. The kinase uses the receptor itself as its main substrate, and there is some evidence that suggests that the receptor could be its only physiologically relevant substrate. Most evidence acquired to date suggests that the tyrosine kinase activity of the receptor is required for transmission of the signal. This has been confirmed by site-directed mutagensis and antibody studies. Some studies with monoclonal antibodies suggest the opposite, but the descriptions of defects in tyrosine kinase activity in patients with insulin resistance suggest a physiological and pathological relevance for the enzymatic activity.

Many proteins of unknown function can be phosphorylated by the insulin receptor tyrosine kinase, but the question in all these cases is which one is relevant. An interesting candidate could be a guanine-nucleotide-binding protein, otherwise known as G proteins. It has been suggested that a G protein is involved in insulin action. The existence of the G_{ins} protein has been suggested by studies on the regulation by insulin of the activity of adenylate cyclase and cAMP phosphodiesterase in liver. Much of the data cannot be explained unless the existence of an insulin-specific G protein is invoked. Unfortunately, G_{ins} has not been purified or characterized and thus it is difficult to take a side on the issue.

Most hormones exert their actions through one of two second-messenger systems. Some hormones, in addition, utilize ion channels as part of the way in which they communicate their signals. Thus, a major step in any signalling system is the generation of a second messenger, but the identity of this molecule remains unknown for insulin. While some of the effects of insulin can be ascribed to alterations in the content of cAMP, insulin does not exclusively act via inhibition of adenylate cyclase or activation of cAMP phosphodiesterase. Similarly, insulin does not act via changes in the content of inositol trisphosphate ($Insl,4,5P_3$). However, insulin does cause a transient increase in diacylglycerol (DG). This observation is of great interest for it suggests that either insulin is capable of stimulating the *de novo* pathway for the synthesis of DG in a very short space of time (less than a minute would be required), or insulin is causing the hydrolysis of a phospholipid other than phosphatidylinositol 4,5-bisphosphate (the precursor for $Insl,4,5P_3$ and DG).

In the last few years there has been considerable excitement concerning the proposal by Saltiel & Cuatrecasas in 1986 (see reference in Chapter 6) that insulin cleaves the glycosyl phosphatidylinositol (GPI) to generate an inositol phosphoglycan (IPG) and DG. The structure of IPG is still unknown, but this candidate for second messenger for insulin has received more praise than criticism: quite an accomplishment in this field! The biological effects of IPG remain to be fully characterized, but the list is large and the effects have been confirmed by various authors. Historical experience in the area of second messengers for insulin should, however, teach us to suspend judgement until all the required evidence is gathered. In my mind, this must include as a priority the structure of the putative IPG and its confirmation by different laboratories, as well as confirmation of the biological effects of this 'mediator'. Very recent studies suggest that IPG might not be exclusively associated with the mechanism of action of insulin, since it has been suggested that both ACTH and EGF can cause the generation of this moilecule. It would be very exciting if, following confirmation of its structure and activities, the IPG were shown to be as ubiquitous a second messenger as cAMP or $Insl,4,5P_3$ are.

So, can a unifying hypothesis be constructed from this wealth of information? If not a full hypothesis, at least a working framework is possible (Fig. 7.1). The multiple effects of insulin occur in different time-frames, some taking a few minutes and others several hours. It is possible, therefore, that different signalling systems mediate different effects. The phosphorylation of some enzymes in response to insulin may be caused by activation of serine/threonine kinases by the insulin receptor tyrosine kinase. The recent work on the regulation of phosphorylation of ribosomal protein S6 points in that direction (see Chapter 4). Enzyme regulation of dephosphorylation could be the result of second messengers such as IPG. DG could

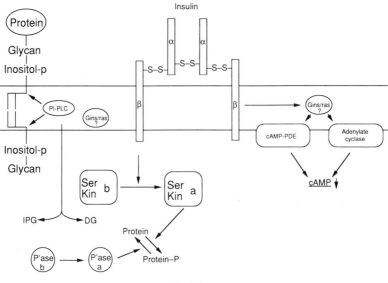

Fig. 7.1.

transiently activate protein kinase C, and lead to protein phosphorylation via that pathway. The activation of an insulin-specific G protein, G_{ins}, could be linked to the inhibition of adenylate cyclase by insulin. The key step in these events is the binding of insulin to its receptors. This in turn would then lead to the activation of a GPl phospholipase C with the subsequent release of 'mediators', as well as the activation of the tyrosine kinase activity.

The picture is getting clearer. The 'black box' theory of insulin action has been substituted for by lighter shades of grey!! We know all the elements in the framework, but we still have to fit the pieces together.

7.2 PERSPECTIVES

What areas of research in insulin action are likely to be of more influence and yield more results in the next few years? Is there any therapeutic potential in any of the current areas of investigation? These are the questions I will briefly cover as part of the final round-up to this work. Obviously, the answers I give are my own opinions of future trends, and it is more than likely that science will contradict most predictions!

A few areas of research appear likely to be the focus of a lot of effort in the near future. The role of the tyrosine kinase activity of the insulin receptor will be further proved through the identification (or lack thereof) of physiologically relevant substrates on the one hand, and by the characterization of phosphotyrosine-specific phosphatases on the other. The existence of a specific phosphatase that would dephosphorylate the insulin receptor would offer a mechanism of regulation of the receptor activity. Since autophosphorylation of the insulin receptor is a required event in signal transmission, modulation of the activity of such a phosphatase would offer a potential site for pharmacological intervention. Inhibitors of the phosphatase could lead to activation of the signalling pathway, a process which could have a therapeutic role in insulin resistance.

An area that seems likely to increase in research effort and which could have an exciting potential is that of examining the role of serine phosphorylation in the molecular mechanisms of insulin action. The identification of a relevant physiological role for serine phosphorylation, and of the cascade of events leading to it, could also result in the identification of further targets for pharmacological intervention. Furthermore, this area may provide a description of the links between insulin binding to its receptor and the cellular events resulting thereby.

Of all the areas of investigation currently underway on insulin action, perhaps the one requiring most critical study is that of the second messengers. As I discussed in Chapter 6, the identification of the structure of the putative second messenger for insulin, as well as the confirmation by different laboratories of its biological effects and its existence, is a major requirement. If all those things prove positive, then a 'mediator' actually has a strong potential as a site of therapeutic intervention. Firstly, compounds that mimic its effects would be of great use, as well as inhibitors of its breakdown or activators of its synthesis. The identification of the enzymes involved in the synthesis and breakdown would therefore be a great advance in this area.

So far, I have discussed only the intracellular side of insulin action. The extracellular events should also require our attention. The identification of the precise site of insulin binding to its receptor will be the next major step in the receptor field. This will also represent a major advance which could lead to the possibility of pharmacological manipulation. Various research groups are currently working on attempting to map the precise amino acid residues within the α-subunit of the insulin receptor to which the hormone binds. This offers enormous possibilities for conformational studies and hence could be therapeutic potential.

Although I discussed in Chapter 2 the regulation of insulin secretion and of insulin gene expression, I will not focus on these areas, since they are more relevant to type I diabetes, and less related to the mechanism of action of insulin.

The next few years are going to offer the clarification of the pieces of the puzzle missing so far. When the mechanism of action of insulin is fully understood, therapeutic intervention will be possible at different sites and will be based more on physiological reality than on random chance.

REFERENCE

Espinal, J. (1987) *Nature* **328**, 574–575.

Index